W9-DCH-853

# Enhancing
# DATA SYSTEMS
## to Improve the Quality of
# CANCER Care

Maria Hewitt and Joseph V. Simone, *Editors*

National Cancer Policy Board

INSTITUTE OF MEDICINE
and
COMMISSION ON LIFE SCIENCES,
NATIONAL RESEARCH COUNCIL

NATIONAL ACADEMY PRESS
Washington, D.C.

NATIONAL ACADEMY PRESS • 2101 Constitution Avenue, N.W. • Washington, DC 20418

NOTICE: The project that is the subject of this report was approved by the Governing Board of the National Research Council, whose members are drawn from the councils of the National Academy of Sciences, the National Academy of Engineering, and the Institute of Medicine. The members of the Board responsible for the report were chosen for their special competences and with regard for appropriate balance.

Support for this project was provided by the National Cancer Institute; the Centers for Disease Control and Prevention; the American Cancer Society; American Society of Clinical Oncology; Amgen, Inc.; Abbott Laboratories; and Hoechst Marion Roussel, Inc. The views presented in this report are those of the Institute of Medicine National Cancer Policy Board and are not necessarily those of the funding agencies.

**International Standard Book No. 0-309-07191-7**

Additional copies of this report are available for sale from the National Academy Press, 2101 Constitution Avenue, N.W., Box 285, Washington, D.C. 20055. Call (800) 624-6242 or (202) 334-3313 (in the Washington metropolitan area), or visit the NAP's home page at **www.nap.edu.** The full text of this report is available at **www.nap.edu.**

For more information about the Institute of Medicine, visit the IOM home page at **www.iom.edu.**

Copyright 2000 by the National Academy of Sciences. All rights reserved.

Printed in the United States of America.

The serpent has been a symbol of long life, healing, and knowledge among almost all cultures and religions since the beginning of recorded history. The serpent adopted as a logotype by the Institute of Medicine is a relief carving from ancient Greece, now held by the Staatliche Museen in Berlin.

*"Knowing is not enough; we must apply.
Willing is not enough; we must do."*
—Goethe

# INSTITUTE OF MEDICINE

Shaping the Future for Health

# THE NATIONAL ACADEMIES

National Academy of Sciences
National Academy of Engineering
Institute of Medicine
National Research Council

The **National Academy of Sciences** is a private, nonprofit, self-perpetuating society of distinguished scholars engaged in scientific and engineering research, dedicated to the furtherance of science and technology and to their use for the general welfare. Upon the authority of the charter granted to it by the Congress in 1863, the Academy has a mandate that requires it to advise the federal government on scientific and technical matters. Dr. Bruce M. Alberts is president of the National Academy of Sciences.

The **National Academy of Engineering** was established in 1964, under the charter of the National Academy of Sciences, as a parallel organization of outstanding engineers. It is autonomous in its administration and in the selection of its members, sharing with the National Academy of Sciences the responsibility for advising the federal government. The National Academy of Engineering also sponsors engineering programs aimed at meeting national needs, encourages education and research, and recognizes the superior achievements of engineers. Dr. William A. Wulf is president of the National Academy of Engineering.

The **Institute of Medicine** was established in 1970 by the National Academy of Sciences to secure the services of eminent members of appropriate professions in the examination of policy matters pertaining to the health of the public. The Institute acts under the responsibility given to the National Academy of Sciences by its congressional charter to be an adviser to the federal government and, upon its own initiative, to identify issues of medical care, research, and education. Dr. Kenneth I. Shine is president of the Institute of Medicine.

The **National Research Council** was organized by the National Academy of Sciences in 1916 to associate the broad community of science and technology with the Academy's purposes of furthering knowledge and advising the federal government. Functioning in accordance with general policies determined by the Academy, the Council has become the principal operating agency of both the National Academy of Sciences and the National Academy of Engineering in providing services to the government, the public, and the scientific and engineering communities. The Council is administered jointly by both Academies and the Institute of Medicine. Dr. Bruce M. Alberts and Dr. William A. Wulf are chairman and vice chairman, respectively, of the National Research Council.

## NATIONAL CANCER POLICY BOARD

**ARNOLD LEVINE** (*Chair*), President, The Rockefeller University

**JOSEPH SIMONE** (*Vice Chair*), Medical Director, Huntsman Cancer Foundation and Institute, University of Utah, Salt Lake City

**ELLEN STOVALL** (*Vice Chair*), Executive Director, National Coalition for Cancer Survivorship, Silver Spring, MD

**DIANA PETITTI** (*Vice Chair*), Director, Research and Evaluation, Kaiser Permanente of Southern California, Pasadena

**TIM BYERS,** Professor of Epidemiology and Program Leader, Clinical Cancer Prevention and Control, University of Colorado Health Sciences Center

**VIVIEN CHEN,** Epidemiology Section Chief and Professor, Louisiana State University Medical Center, New Orleans

**SUSAN CURRY,** Director, Center for Health Studies, Group Health Cooperative of Puget Sound, Seattle

**NORMAN DANIELS,** Professor of Philosophy, Tufts University

**KATHLEEN FOLEY,** Chief, Pain Service, Department of Neurology, Memorial Sloan-Kettering Cancer Center, New York City

**THOMAS KELLY,** Boury Professor and Chairman, Department of Molecular Biology and Genetics, Johns Hopkins University School of Medicine

**MARK McCLELLAN,** Assistant Professor of Economics, Stanford University

**WILLIAM McGUIRE,** Chief Executive Officer, UnitedHealth Group, Minnetonka, MN

**JOHN MENDELSOHN,** President, University of Texas M.D. Anderson Cancer Center, Houston

**MONICA MORROW,** Professor of Surgery and Director, Lynn Sage Comprehensive Breast Program, Northwestern University Medical School

**NANCY MUELLER,** Professor of Epidemiology, Harvard School of Public Health

**PILAR OSSORIO,** Assistant Professor of Law and Medical Ethics, and Associate Director for Programming, Center for the Study of Race and Ethnicity in Medicine, University of Wisconsin Law School, Madison

**CECIL PICKETT,** Executive Vice President of Discovery Research, Schering-Plough Research Institute, Kenilworth, NJ

**JOHN SEFFRIN,** Chief Executive Officer, American Cancer Society, Atlanta

**SANDRA UNDERWOOD,** American Cancer Society Oncology Nursing Professor and Professor, Health Maintenance Department, University of Wisconsin School of Nursing, Milwaukee

**FRANCES VISCO,** President, National Breast Cancer Coalition, Washington, DC

**SUSAN WEINER,** President, The Children's Cause, Silver Spring, MD

We also wish to thank former board members **Peter Howley, John Bailar, Jospeph Davie, Robert Day,** and **Jane Sisk** for their contributions to the development of this report during their term of service on the board.

**Staff**

**MARIA HEWITT,** Study Director

**ROBERT COOK-DEEGAN,** Director, National Cancer Policy Board (through August 2000)

**CARMIE CHAN,** Research Assistant

**ROGER HERDMAN,** Director, National Cancer Policy Board (from September 2000)

**ELLEN JOHNSON,** Administrative Assistant

# Acknowledgments

This report brings together the diverse fields of health services research, cancer surveillance, and informatics, and the authors relied heavily upon the contributions of many people with expertise in these areas. Our goal in preparing this report was to address pressing issues related to improving the quality of cancer care, while staying focused on the technicalities of data systems and processes needed to further these quality-related goals. We consulted extensively with experts in the many disciplines covered in this report and are deeply indebted to them.

This report emanates from the National Cancer Policy Board (board). The board has a wide range of expertise in, for example, basic research, clinical practice, administration, and patient advocacy. For this report, the board's expertise was augmented by outside experts. Many of these experts were assembled at a workshop in October 1999 at The National Academies to present relevant papers and participate in discussions with the board (see the workshop agenda and list of participants in Appendix B). The board is particularly indebted to Thomas Smith for preparing the charge to the workshop and for his dynamic leadership of the workshop. The entire board active in 1999 was involved in this report's development, but the authors want particularly to thank four members who made significant contributions: Vivien Chen, Monica Morrow, Diana Petitti, and Jane Sisk. Members of the Board, Arnold Levine, Tim Byers, Mark McClellan, Nancy Mueller, Cecil Pickett, and Susan Weiner, could not participate in this report because they were appointed after it was completed. The report benefited greatly from the inclusion of 10 case studies illustrating how pioneers in monitoring the quality of cancer care are using existing data within their practices or systems of care. We are very grateful to David Lansky of the Foundation for Accountability for helping us identify some of these programs. We would especially like to thank the following individuals for the time and effort they contributed in completing these case studies (listed in order of presentation in the report):

1.  Peter Eisenberg, Marin Oncology Associates;
2.  Grant Swanson, Kimberly Bergstrom, and Roger Shiffman, OnCare;
3.  Jean Owen, American College of Radiology;
4.  Gale Katterhagen, Sutter Health Breast Cancer Quality Project;
5.  Laurie Skokan, Providence Health System;
6.  Jane Weeks, National Comprehensive Cancer Network;
7.  Stephen Edge, Roswell Park Cancer Institute;
8.  Tim Byers, Colorado Medicare beneficiaries case study;
9.  Becky J. Cherney, Central Florida Health Care Coalition; and
10. Monica Morrow, National Cancer Data Base.

Kevin Brady, Mary Kaeser, and Dan Miller at the Centers for Disease Control and Prevention (CDC) provided valuable assistance with our review of the National Program of Cancer Registries. Staff at the National Cancer Institute (NCI) were very helpful in providing relevant materials and reviewing sections of the report describing NCI-sponsored programs and research. A special thanks goes to Rachael Ballard-Barbash, Martin Brown, Brenda Edwards, Linda Harlan, Arnold Potosky, and Joan Warren.

The document benefited greatly from an open, technical review at the January 5, 2000, board meeting. Here, invited experts had an opportunity to critique an early draft of the report and engage in discussions with the board. Our invited experts included: Joseph Bailes, American Society of Clinical Oncology; Christopher Desch, Medical College of Virginia, Virginia Commonwealth University; Robert Hiatt, Rachel Ballard-Barbash, and Joseph Lipscomb, Division of Cancer Control and Population Sciences, NCI; Nancy Lee, Division of Cancer Prevention and Control, National Center for Chronic Disease Prevention and Health Promotion, Centers for Disease Control; Mitchell Morris, M.D. Anderson Cancer Center; Jean Owen, American College of Radiology; Nancy Riese Daly, American Society for Therapeutic Radiology and Oncology; Edward Sondik, National Center for Health Statistics; Thomas Tucker, University of Kentucky; and Jane Weeks, Dana-Farber Cancer Institute.

Board staff were essential to completing this report. Robert Cook-Deegan, the board director, helped develop the open review process and reviewed drafts. Hellen Gelband provided helpful suggestions to improve the draft document. As research assistant throughout the study, Carmie Chan was resourceful and thorough as she located references and completed tables for appendices. Ellen Johnson, the project administrative assistant, was invaluable in planning the workshop, steering the report through Academy procedures, and supporting the board.

A number of quality-related projects conducted within the Health Care Services Division of the Institute of Medicine (IOM) provided very important background information for the report, especially in the areas of informatics and computer-based patient records.

## REVIEWERS

This report has been reviewed in draft form by individuals chosen for their diverse perspectives and technical expertise, in accordance with procedures approved by the National Research Council's Report Review Committee. The purpose of this independent review is to provide candid and critical comments that will assist the Institute of Medicine and the National Research Council in making the published report as sound as possible and to ensure that the report meets institutional standards for objectivity, evidence, and responsiveness to the study charge. The review comments and the draft manuscript remain confidential to protect the integrity of the deliberative process.

The National Cancer Policy Board wishes to thank the following individuals for their participation in the review of this report:

**David J. Ballard,** Senior Vice President, Health Care Research and Improvement, Baylor Health Care System, Dallas, TX

**Paul Clayton,** Intermountain Health Care, Salt Lake City, UT

**Holly Howe,** Executive Director, National Association of Centralized Cancer Care Registries, Springfield, IL

**David Lansky,** The Foundation for Accountability, Portland, OR

**Elizabeth McGlynn,** RAND Corporation, Health Sciences Program, Santa Monica, CA

**Ann B. Nattinger,** Department of Medicine, Medical College of Wisconsin

**Edward B. Perrin,** Professor, Emeritus, Department of Health Services, University of Washington

Although the individuals acknowledged have provided valuable comments and suggestions, responsibility for the final contents of the report rests solely with the National Cancer Policy Board, the Institute of Medicine, and the National Research Council.

# Contents

EXECUTIVE SUMMARY ............................................................................ 1

1   INTRODUCTION .................................................................................. 8
    Role of the National Cancer Policy Board, 8
    Framework of the Report, 10

2   WHAT WOULD AN IDEAL CANCER CARE DATA SYSTEM
    LOOK LIKE? ...................................................................................... 11
    Well-Established Quality-of-Care Measures, 12
    Computer-Based Patient Records, 14
    Standard Reporting, 14
    National, Population-Based Case Selection, 15
    Repeated Studies to Monitor National Trends, 16
    Established Benchmarks for Quality Improvement, 16
    Data Systems for Local Quality Assurance Purposes, 16
    Public Reporting of Selected Aggregate Quality Scores, 17
    Adaptability, 17
    Protections to Assure Privacy of Health Information, 17

3   HOW ARE HEALTHCARE SYSTEMS MONITORING
    QUALITY TODAY? ............................................................................. 18
    Case Studies—Illustrations of the Use of Data to Monitor Cancer Care
        Quality, 18
    Summary, 34

**4    THE DATA INFRASTRUCTURE FOR HEALTH SERVICES
      RESEARCH** ................................................................................ 37
      Linkage of Cancer Registries to Administrative Data, 37
      Cancer Registries as a Sampling Frame for Special Studies, 39
      Developing Health Services Research Consortiums, 42
      Federal Health Surveys and Data, 43
      Summary, 45

**5    STATUS OF THE CANCER CARE DATA SYSTEM** ........................ 46
      Well-Established Quality-of-Care Measures, 47
      Computer-Based Patient Records, 52
      Standard Reporting, 53
      National, Population-Based Case Selection, 55
      Established Benchmarks for Quality Improvement, 63
      Data Systems for Local Quality Assurance Purposes, 66
      Summary, 75

**6    FINDINGS AND RECOMMENDATIONS** ......................................... 76
      What Would the Ideal Cancer Care Data System Look Like? 77
      How Are Current Cancer Data Systems Meeting the Needs of
          Healthcare Systems? 78
      What Steps Can be Taken to Enhance Data Systems So That They Can Be
          Used to Monitor and Improve the Quality of Cancer Care? 82

**REFERENCES** ................................................................................. 95

**ACRONYMS AND ABBREVIATIONS** ....................................... 105

**APPENDIXES**
A    *Ensuring Quality Cancer Care,* Report Summary, 109
B    Workshop Agenda and Participants, 123
C    Summary of Selected Registry-Based Quality Studies, 131
D    Information on Cancer Registries, by State, 141
E    Reporting Requirements, NPCR, NCDB, SEER, 148

**INDEX** ............................................................................................ 155

# Executive Summary

The National Cancer Policy Board (board) concluded in its April 1999 report, *Ensuring Quality Cancer Care*, that based on the best available evidence, some individuals with cancer do not receive care known to be effective for their condition. The magnitude of the problem is not known, but the board believes it is substantial (IOM 1999a). Why do we know so little about the nature and extent of care-related problems that affect so many Americans? In part, the lack of knowledge is a result of the fragmented nature of health care in the United States, with no central point of accountability. There are also more technical reasons, for example, an absence until recently of valid indicators of the quality of care, and the lack of comprehensive data systems with which to measure quality.

Data systems are the backbone of efforts to improve the quality of health care. Performance data can provide the impetus for providers, health plans, and systems of care to change. Experience suggests that quality within health systems can improve when organizations measure and monitor performance, encourage change through incentive systems and education, and hold providers accountable to the quality expectations of purchasers and consumers. Data systems can also help gauge the status of cancer care across the nation, alerting political, professional, and advocacy leaders to the need for action. An active health services research community furthers quality improvement by using data systems to determine correlates of quality cancer care and to elucidate the reasons for poor quality care.

Quality assessment studies should ideally include recently diagnosed individuals with cancer in care settings representative of contemporary practice across the country and rely on information sources in sufficient detail to allow

1

sound analyses (IOM, 1999a). Despite investments by federal, state, and private groups in cancer-related data systems, there are gaps in the availability of data needed to conduct quality-of-care studies, redundancies in data collection, and problems with the completeness, timeliness, and quality of the data that are collected. At the same time, there are tremendous opportunities to improve cancer care data systems through:

- movement toward a comprehensive and coordinated national system,
- leadership within the cancer care community,
- cooperation among groups providing cancer data,
- integration with national efforts to further quality of care, and
- the application of new information technologies (e.g., computer-based patient records, Internet communications).

The board held a workshop in October 1999 to establish the characteristics of an ideal cancer care data system and to identify financial and other resources needed to help achieve that ideal. This report summarizes the workshop proceedings and board deliberations, then presents the board's recommendations for steps that can be taken to enhance current data systems to improve cancer care. The report addresses three questions:

1. What would the ideal cancer care data system look like?
2. How are current cancer data systems meeting the needs of healthcare systems?
3. What steps can be taken to enhance data systems so that they can be used to monitor and improve the quality of cancer care?

## WHAT WOULD THE IDEAL CANCER CARE
## DATA SYSTEM LOOK LIKE?

The board concluded that to meet national quality-of-care objectives, an ideal cancer care data system (which could include several distinct databases) would have the following 10 attributes:

1. *A set of well-established quality-of-care measures*—a single core set of quality measures must be developed, using the best available evidence for the full spectrum of an individual's care—from early detection to palliative and end-of-life care.

2. *Reliance on computer-based patient records for information on patient care and outcomes*—adoption of information technology can improve the timeliness and accuracy of information on the quality of cancer care.

3. *Standard reporting of cancer stage, presence of coexisting disease (i.e., comorbidity), and processes of care*—national quality assessments depend on the uniform recording of data elements needed to accurately assess care.

4. *National, population-based case selection*—complete ascertainment of incident cancer cases by cancer registries is a prerequisite for national quality assessments, allowing case selection for studies whose results can be generalized to the total population and assessments of quality for important subgroups—for example, individuals of low socioeconomic status and individuals enrolled in certain types of health plans or delivery systems.

5. *Repeated cross sectional studies to monitor national trends*—a series of measures is needed to monitor progress over time.

6. *Established benchmarks for quality improvement*—systems of care need information on accepted standards of care (e.g., clinical practice guidelines) with which to assess their performance.

7. *Data systems for internal quality assurance purposes*—systems of care need internal data to monitor performance and quality improvement.

8. *Public reporting of selected aggregate quality scores*—quality measures enable consumers and purchasers to judge the quality of a system of care by its performance relative to evidence-based standards.

9. *Adaptability*—new evidence on quality measures, changes in healthcare delivery, and technological innovation are among the factors that necessitate flexibility in data systems.

10. *Privacy protections*—legal protections and data security systems must be in place to ensure that data collected and stored about an individual's diagnosis and treatment of cancer are used only for legitimate purposes.

## HOW ARE CURRENT CANCER DATA SYSTEMS MEETING THE NEEDS OF HEALTHCARE SYSTEMS?

The board's review of current cancer care data systems suggests that we are far from the ideal. Relatively few healthcare systems are monitoring the quality of cancer care. Serious barriers impeding such efforts include:

- a lack of recognized measures of quality;
- an absence of benchmarks with which to measure progress and success;
- reliance on hospital-based data retrieval, while cancer care is shifting to ambulatory care settings;
- reliance on retrospective medical chart reviews for data, a method that is labor intensive, inefficient, and prone to error relative to the prospective electronic capture of information possible through computer-based patient record systems;
- methodologic difficulties (e.g., adequacy of sample sizes for comparison, availability of data with which to control for differences in patient mix); and
- concerns about protecting the privacy and confidentiality of patient information.

Advances in information technology and the evolution of fully integrated systems of care may ultimately resolve some of the problems associated with existing data systems. Computer-based patient records and electronic communication have the potential to greatly improve the quality, comprehensiveness, and timeliness of data. And data systems built to meet the needs of disease management programs could capture information on an individual's full episode of care, regardless of where in the system care was provided. Such developments are, however, likely years away from widespread application and are in part dependent on resolving policy issues concerning the maintenance of confidentiality of patient information.

In the short term, three national cancer-related databases hold great promise to further quality improvement efforts:

1. the National Program of Cancer Registries (NPCR) of the Centers for Disease Control and Prevention (CDC);
2. the Surveillance, Epidemiology, and End Results (SEER) program of the National Cancer Institute (NCI); and
3. the National Cancer Data Base (NCDB), sponsored by the American College of Surgeon's Commission on Cancer (ACoS-CoC) and the American Cancer Society.

NPCR and SEER are cancer surveillance systems with a primary mission of providing population-based estimates with which to understand the occurrence and distribution of cancer. These surveillance systems can also become powerful tools for assessing quality of care when linked to other data sources or when used to select individual cases for special studies. Surveillance databases have great potential to provide population-based estimates of quality-of-care problems. Despite the value of these databases, sustaining them is difficult, let alone expanding their use for quality measurement. Most states do not have the resources to augment their current workload to conduct studies of quality care, which fall outside their primary mission of cancer surveillance; many states struggle merely to ensure that basic cancer surveillance continues.

The ACoS-CoC and the American Cancer Society have long supported the examination of quality of cancer care through the most extensive national data collection effort dedicated to this purpose, NCDB. NCDB has tremendous potential to provide detailed information regarding quality to the facilities that report to it, thereby encouraging improvements in performance. As a source of national information on quality, however, NCDB has limitations because of its lack of complete coverage. Only facilities with cancer programs approved by ACoS-CoC must report data to NCDB, and most of these are hospitals. Cases that tend to be missed in NCDB are those diagnosed and treated in unapproved facilities and ambulatory care settings. While NCDB is not nationally representative, estimates are that roughly 80 percent of incident cancer cases are reported to NCDB, making it a powerful resource for internal quality assessments within sites of cancer care serving the majority of Americans.

Of all available systems, NCDB includes the most extensive set of treatment-related items. NPCR and SEER include first course treatment, but little else. Gathering data on chemotherapy and adjuvant radiation therapy is challenging because the individuals collecting much of the data for data systems, cancer registrars, are generally hospital based. They abstract needed information from the hospital chart. Procedures occurring outside of the hospital (e.g., in community-based, private practice office settings) are usually not recorded in the hospital chart, and because there are generally insufficient resources to track such care, treatment data from cancer registries and databases is often too incomplete to use for quality studies.

## WHAT STEPS CAN BE TAKEN TO ENHANCE DATA SYSTEMS SO THAT THEY CAN BE USED TO MONITOR AND IMPROVE THE QUALITY OF CANCER CARE?

The board recommends that steps be taken in three areas to improve the quality of cancer care:

1. Enhance key elements of the data system infrastructure: quality-of-care measures, cancer registries and databases, data collection technologies, and analytic capacity.
2. Expand support for analyses of quality of cancer care using existing data systems.
3. Monitor the effectiveness of data systems to promote quality improvement within health systems.

### 1. Enhance Key Elements of the Data System Infrastructure

**Recommendation 1: Develop a core set of cancer care quality measures.**

**a. The secretary of the Department of Health and Human Services (DHHS) should designate a committee made up of representatives of public institutions (e.g., the DHHS Quality of Cancer Care Committee, state cancer registries, academic institutions) and private groups (e.g., consumer organizations, professional associations, purchasers, health insurers and plans) to: 1) identify a single core set of quality measures that span the full spectrum of an individual's care and are based on the best available evidence; 2) advise other national groups (e.g., National Committee for Quality Assurance, Joint Commission for the Accreditation of Healthcare Organizations, Quality Forum) to adopt the recommended core set**

of measures; and 3) monitor the progress of ongoing efforts to improve standard reporting of cancer stage and comorbidity.

b. Research sponsors (e.g., Agency for Healthcare Research and Quality [AHRQ], National Cancer Institute [NCI], Health Care Financing Administration [HCFA], Department of Veterans Affairs [VA]) should invest in studies to identify evidence-based quality indicators across the continuum of cancer care.

c. Ongoing efforts to standardize reporting of cancer stage and comorbidity should receive a high priority and be fully supported.

d. Efforts to identify quality of cancer care measures should be coordinated with ongoing national efforts regarding quality of care.

Recommendation 2: Congress should increase support to the Centers for Disease Control and Prevention (CDC) for the National Program of Cancer Registries (NPCR) to improve the capacity of states to achieve complete coverage and timely reporting of incident cancer cases. NPCR's primary purpose is cancer surveillance, but NPCR, together with SEER, has great potential to facilitate national, population-based assessments of the quality of cancer care through linkage studies and by serving as a sample frame for special studies.

Recommendation 3: Private cancer-related organizations should join the American Cancer Society and the American College of Surgeons' to provide financial support for the National Cancer Data Base. Expanded support would facilitate efforts underway to report quality benchmarks and performance data to institutions providing cancer care.

Recommendation 4: Federal research agencies (e.g., NCI, CDC, AHRQ, HCFA) should support research and demonstration projects to identify new mechanisms to organize and finance the collection of data for cancer care quality studies. Current data systems tend to be hospital based, while cancer care is shifting to outpatient settings. New models are needed to capture entire episodes of care, irrespective of the setting of care.

Recommendation 5: Federal research agencies (e.g., National Institutes of Health [NIH], Food and Drug Administration [FDA], CDC, and VA) should support public-private partnerships to develop technologies, including computer-based patient record systems and intranet-based communication systems, that will improve the availability, quality, and timeliness of clinical data relevant to assessing quality of cancer care.

**Recommendation 6:** Federal research agencies (e.g., NCI, AHRQ, VA) should expand support for training in health services research and training of professionals with expertise in the measurement of quality of care and the implementation and evaluation of interventions designed to improve the quality of care.

## 2. Expand Support for Analyses of Quality of Cancer Care Using Existing Data Systems

**Recommendation 7:** Federal research agencies (e.g., NCI, AHRQ, VA) should expand support for health services research, especially studies based on the linkage of cancer registry to administrative data and special studies of cases sampled from cancer registries. Resources should also be made available through NPCR and SEER to provide technical assistance to states to help them expand the capability of using cancer registry data for quality improvement initiatives. NPCR should also be supported in its efforts to consolidate state data and link them to national data files.

**Recommendation 8:** Federal research agencies (e.g., NCI, AHRQ, HCFA) should develop models for the conduct of linkage studies and the release of confidential data for research purposes that protect the confidentiality and privacy of healthcare information.

## 3. Monitor the Effectiveness of Data Systems to Promote Quality Improvement Within Health Systems.

**Recommendation 9:** Federal research agencies (e.g., NCI, AHRQ, HCFA, VA) should fund demonstration projects to assess the application of quality monitoring programs within healthcare systems and the impact of data-driven changes in the delivery of services on the quality of health care. Findings from the demonstrations should be disseminated widely to consumers, payers, purchasers, and cancer care providers.

# 1

# Introduction

The National Cancer Policy Board (hereafter, the board) concluded in its April 1999 report, *Ensuring Quality Cancer Care,* that based on the best available evidence, some individuals with cancer do not receive care known to be effective for their condition. The magnitude of the problem is not known, but the NCPB believes it is substantial (IOM, 1999a). Why do we know so little about the nature and extent of care-related problems that affect so many Americans? In part, the lack of knowledge is a result of the fragmented nature of the American healthcare system, which has no central point of accountability. There are also more technical reasons, for example, an absence until recently of valid indicators of the quality of care and the lack of comprehensive data systems with which to measure quality.

## ROLE OF THE NATIONAL CANCER POLICY BOARD

The board was established in March 1997 at the Institute of Medicine (IOM) and National Research Council to address issues that arise in the prevention, control, diagnosis, treatment, and palliation of cancer. The 20-member board includes healthcare consumers, providers, and investigators in several disciplines (see membership roster). In April 1999, the board released a report, *Ensuring Quality Cancer Care,* which:

- described important elements of the current cancer care "system," from early detection to end-of-life care, in the context of the rapidly changing healthcare environment;

- identified major barriers that impede access to quality cancer care;
- defined quality cancer care and described its measurement;
- provided examples of problems that limit early detection, accurate diagnosis, optimal treatment, and responsive supportive care;
- reviewed and critiqued systems of accountability that are in place to help ensure the receipt of quality cancer care;
- assessed whether ongoing cancer-related health services research is addressing outstanding questions about the quality of cancer care; and
- presented recommendations to enhance cancer care for consideration by Congress, public and private healthcare purchasers, health plans, individual consumers, healthcare providers, and researchers (see report summary in Appendix A).

The board found that it was difficult to judge the quality of contemporary cancer care practice from available sources because of:

- a lack of current data (i.e., many published studies rely on the experience of patients diagnosed and treated in the 1980s),
- limited information on the care experience across geographic areas and sites of care, and
- methodological shortcomings (e.g., a lack of control for important clinical characteristics, such as the presence of diseases other than cancer).

The board concluded that a cancer data system is needed that can provide quality benchmarks for use by systems of care (e.g., hospitals, provider groups, and managed care systems). An ideal data system would include recently diagnosed individuals with cancer in care settings representative of contemporary practice across the country, using information sources with sufficient detail to allow appropriate comparisons. The board, recognizing that current data systems and quality assessments were far from this ideal, held a workshop in October 1999 to:

- identify how best to meet the data needs for cancer in light of quality monitoring goals,
- identify financial and other resources needed to improve the cancer data system to achieve quality-related goals, and
- develop strategies to improve data available on the quality of cancer care.

This report summarizes the workshop proceedings and board deliberations, then presents the board's recommendations for action (see workshop agenda and list of participants in Appendix B). The report addresses three questions:

1. What would the ideal cancer care data system look like?

2. How are current cancer data systems meeting the needs of healthcare systems?

3. What steps can be taken to enhance data systems so that they can be used to monitor and improve the quality of cancer care?

This report focuses on enhancing current cancer-related data systems and supplements the board's earlier work, *Ensuring Quality Cancer Care* (IOM, 1999a). Other work at IOM takes a broader approach to healthcare data systems and quality reporting. A committee has recently been formed at IOM to design a national quality report to provide information on the quality of care provided by the U.S. healthcare industry (see "National Quality Report on Health Care Delivery" under "Ongoing Studies," Board on Health Care Services, at www.iom. edu). A 1999 workshop (see Appendix B) addressed how information technology can be used to improve quality in health care. Other IOM publications have addressed the measurement of healthcare quality (IOM, 1999b) and advances in computer-based patient records (IOM, 1997).

## FRAMEWORK OF THE REPORT

**Chapter 2** describes the attributes of an ideal data system for cancer care quality monitoring.

**Chapter 3** illustrates, through a series of case studies, ways in which providers, hospitals, health plans, and healthcare purchasers are using available data to assess the quality of cancer care.

**Chapter 4** summarizes the data infrastructure for health services research.

**Chapter 5** discusses important elements of a national cancer data system and how the current data system matches the ideal system.

**Chapter 6** summarizes the report findings and presents the board's recommendations.

# 2

# What Would an Ideal Cancer Care Data System Look Like?

The United States has no national cancer care data system. Like the U.S. healthcare system, the data systems available to assess the quality of care on a national or regional basis are fragmented (Pollock and Rice, 1997). Advancing quality of care involves applying data in at least three ways:

- assessing levels and trends in quality of care for whole populations (e.g., the nation, by region, by state) or important subgroups (e.g., racial/ethnic groups, the medically uninsured) to identify the magnitude of quality problems and their distribution,
- determining correlates of quality cancer care (e.g., characteristics of patients and health systems) to elucidate potential causal factors, and
- measuring and monitoring the quality of cancer care within systems of care to promote quality improvement and allow purchasers and the public to hold systems and providers accountable for the care they deliver.

Available databases have been creatively exploited to meet these objectives, but most sources can be critiqued on one of two important grounds—a lack of geographic representation, or the absence of critical data elements needed to adjust results to make comparisons. To put the limitations of current data systems in perspective, this chapter describes what might be construed as an ideal cancer care data system. Later, in Chapter 5, the application of current data systems for quality monitoring is assessed in the context of this ideal.

The board concluded that to meet national quality-of-care objectives, a cancer care data system (which could include several distinct databases) would have the following 10 attributes:

1. a set of well-established quality-of-care measures,
2. reliance on computer-based patient records for information on patient care and outcomes,
3. standard reporting of cancer stage, comorbidity, and processes of care,
4. national, population-based case selection,
5. repeated cross-sectional studies to monitor national trends,
6. established benchmarks for quality improvement,
7. data systems for local quality assurance purposes,
8. public reporting of selected aggregate quality scores,
9. adaptability, and
10. protections to ensure privacy of health information.

## WELL-ESTABLISHED QUALITY-OF-CARE MEASURES

At the foundation of an ideal cancer care data system would be a single core set of well-established, "evidence-based" quality measures for the full spectrum of an individual's care—from early detection, to palliation, to end-of-life care. Most measures would be of "processes of care" known through clinical trial research to improve outcomes. Such measures are well suited to quality assessment because if performance falls short, it is clear what needs to be done (i.e., intervene to change process of care). A process measure might identify:

- overuse of tests or procedures with no known efficacy (e.g., use of bone scans following primary therapy for breast cancer to detect secondary cancer),
- underuse of tests or procedures known to be effective (e.g., use of radiation therapy following lumpectomy for breast cancer), and
- misuse of interventions (e.g., too low a dose of chemotherapy).

Criteria for evaluating quality measures include: that they are clinically meaningful, scientifically sound, and interpretable as judged by the intended audience (IOM, 1999b; McGlynn, 1998). How robust a particular indicator is can be judged according to the level of evidence available to support the link between a particular process of care and good outcomes (Box 2.1). Common sense might dictate the use of certain measures, despite their lack of evidence regarding effectiveness. Documentation in the medical chart of cancer stage, for example, could be considered an indicator because it is a prerequisite to developing a treatment plan and must be communicated to providers throughout a patient's care. In addition to meeting standards of evidence (or common sense), measures must be applicable in practice settings. In certain care settings, for example, there may be too few patients available for statistically valid comparisons.

---

**BOX 2.1  Levels of Evidence Applied to Clinical Research**

The "hierarchy of evidence" applied to clinical research (i.e., when the question is whether a given treatment is effective in patients with a specific type of cancer) is well established and agreed upon. The following version is taken from the well-respected U.S. Preventive Services Task Force, proceeding from the most reliable to the least reliable type of evidence (i.e., from grade I to grade III):

I       Evidence obtained from at least one properly randomized controlled trial.

II-1    Evidence obtained from well-designed controlled trials without randomization.

II-2    Evidence obtained from well-designed cohort or case-control studies, preferably from more than one center or research group.

II-3    Evidence obtained from multiple time series with or without the intervention—dramatic results in uncontrolled experiments (e.g., the results of the introduction of penicillin treatment in the 1940s) could also be regarded as this type of evidence.

III     Opinions of respected authorities, based on clinical experience, descriptive studies and case reports, or reports of expert committees.

SOURCE: U.S. Department of Health and Human Services, Office of Public Health and Science, 1996, p. 862.

---

An ideal cancer care data system would also provide information on the healthcare experience of individuals with cancer. Optimally, individuals within the care system would report that their care had been well coordinated, that they had easy communication with their providers, and that they felt their care had been consistent with their personal preferences. The quality of an individual's experience within the cancer care system—whether care was perceived to be well coordinated, respectful, supportive, and compassionate—would be assessed through validated survey instruments.

Measures for which there is suspected variation, or low overall performance, would be selected to assess quality. If adherence to a standard were known to be uniformly high, there would be no good reason to monitor it. And if quality had improved to meet or exceed a target, that measure might be dropped from the indicator set. The measurement set would be a dynamic one, with additional process measures being added as they are identified through research, and old ones dropped as national (or regional) norms reach established targets. Certain key measures could be maintained to allow for analyses of trends.

## COMPUTER-BASED PATIENT RECORDS

In an ideal system, healthcare providers could easily record patient care data using a computer-based patient record (CPR) system. The entry system would be "smart" and prompt providers to adhere to standards for reporting stage, comorbidity, processes of care, and care outcomes (e.g., complications, indicators of quality of life). CPR systems have the capacity to transform patient care and improve quality. Benefits of CPR systems include (IOM, 1997):

- *integrated view of patient data*: patient data are accessible whenever and wherever clinical decisions are made, independent of where the data was originally acquired;
- *access to knowledge resources*: providers can access medical and administrative knowledge at the time decisions are made;
- *physician order entry and clinician data entry*: systems allow proactive influence on physicians' practice patterns;
- *integrated communications support*: activities of healthcare professionals from multiple organizations at different sites can be coordinated;
- *clinical decision support*: prompts regarding clinical guidelines, drug interactions, and abnormal laboratory results can improve the clinician's efficiency and compliance with accepted standards of practice.

With CPRs, healthcare providers would have access to information at the point of care to aid in clinical decision making and patient counseling. For purposes of cancer registration, CPRs could automate the abstraction of necessary data and dramatically improve the timeliness of reporting. Intranets, controlled-access versions of the Internet, could be set up to facilitate data exchange between clinicians and registries.

## STANDARD REPORTING

Outcomes of treatment for cancer vary markedly by stage of illness (a measure of how advanced cancer is) and by the degree to which patients have other diseases or illnesses along with their cancer (called comorbidity). When making comparisons between groups of patients (e.g., comparing surgical outcomes among patients cared for in large versus small hospitals), it is essential to control both for their stage of illness and comorbidity. Without such controls, worse outcomes could be attributed to differences in care, when in reality they are due to differences in the mix of patients in the two types of hospitals. Quality assessments depend on the accurate recording of stage and degree of comorbidity because what is considered appropriate treatment varies by these patient attributes. An ideal cancer care data system would include information on cancer stage and comorbidity, reported in a standard way.

## NATIONAL, POPULATION-BASED CASE SELECTION

Convenience samples are frequently used for quality studies, but the results of such studies are often difficult to interpret because of their limited population coverage. A study of the quality of cancer care conducted in a few states or within a particular health plan, for example, might highlight problems in quality; however, broader inferences from such studies to the care received in other areas or other plans are difficult to make because the population from which the results are drawn usually differs in important ways from the broader population.

The determinants of quality of care have not yet been well established, but evidence suggests the presence of significant geographic variation in patterns of cancer care that persist even after adjustments are made for characteristics of patients and their access to services (Schuster, 1998a). There is much interest in how aspects of healthcare delivery affect the quality of care, and certainly the organization of health care varies markedly by geography. Managed care penetration, for example, is very high in certain states (e.g., California, Minnesota) but extremely low in some states in the South (Modern Healthcare, 1999). Other evidence suggests that certain groups of patients are more prone to poor quality care, for example, individuals of low socioeconomic status and those who lack health insurance coverage. If a quality-of-care study relied on data from areas that differed in sociodemographic make-up from the nation as a whole, results may not accurately reflect the state of quality of care for the nation.

In an ideal study of cancer care quality, each newly identified cancer patient in the United States would have a chance to be in the study, and the probability of inclusion would be known. While this approach sounds simple, it is quite difficult to achieve. It requires having a complete listing of individuals with cancer for a defined geographic area. Because cancer treatment differs so markedly by type and stage of cancer, quality studies are often targeted to specific types and stages of cancer. Some cancers are extremely rare, and complete case ascertainment may be needed to capture an accurate assessment of quality of care. For common cancers, however, careful sampling techniques may be applied to obtain a representative group of patients for study.

Ideally, each state would have accurate, timely reports from all cancer care providers in the state (and from providers out of state who diagnosed a patient residing in that state) so that lists or "frames" could be developed for sampling purposes. Studies designed to be representative of a total population are often referred to as "population-based" studies.

Many concerns about quality care relate to the initial stages of care—diagnosis, treatment, and follow-up care. Studies of these phases of care can rely on samples from among the 1.2 million new cases of cancer expected annually. Other means of patient selection could be used to study the quality of care at the end of life. For this phase of care, prospective studies might be conducted among a cohort of newly diagnosed patients with cancers having high associated mortality, or with samples of seriously ill patients identified in hospitals, nursing homes, or hospices.

The selection of patients for study need not occur at the level of the individual with cancer. If a comprehensive listing of cancer care providers were available, a multistage process of case identification could be used. First, a sample of providers could be selected, then within practices, patients (or a sample of patients) could be selected who met entry criteria.

## REPEATED STUDIES TO MONITOR NATIONAL TRENDS

National studies aimed at assessing the quality of cancer care would ideally be repeated at regular intervals to measure progress toward improvement goals. Just as national surveys are conducted regularly of the general population, healthcare providers, and certain healthcare institutions to monitor the achievement of health objectives for the nation (e.g., Healthy People 2010), so too should there be assessments of the quality of care. Trend data may convey the feasibility of reaching established goals, and variation in rates of change across regions can establish what is achievable within a given space of time.

## ESTABLISHED BENCHMARKS FOR
## QUALITY IMPROVEMENT

If information on processes of care were available on a national sample of recently diagnosed cancer cases, contemporary patterns of cancer care could be described. These national patterns of care data could then be used to assess compliance to accepted standards of care and to establish specific benchmarks, or targets, for the improvement of care. The benchmarks would be set in such a way that they represented excellence, and at the same time would be achievable by practitioners.

## DATA SYSTEMS FOR LOCAL
## QUALITY ASSURANCE PURPOSES

Opportunities to change practice behavior and improve the quality of cancer care rest within local systems of care, for example, hospitals, health plans, and provider groups. The degree to which data can be provided at local levels rests in part on the cancer caseload. For statistically valid comparisons to be made, a sufficient number of individuals with cancer must be present in each site of care; however, data from smaller units can often be aggregated into larger service areas. Alternatively, it is sometimes possible to apply general measures of quality across discrete patient populations. It may be feasible, for example, to apply a general indicator for appropriate use of adjuvant therapy across several types of cancer (e.g., breast, colorectal) or appropriate use of palliative care (e.g., pain management) among individuals with advanced or recurrent cancer.

## PUBLIC REPORTING OF SELECTED
## AGGREGATE QUALITY SCORES

An ideal cancer care data system would allow hospitals and health plans to assess their care relative to national or regional norms and to identify ways that care could be improved. Facilities and plans would receive periodic, easy-to-read charts comparing their recent experience against national or regional norms. For health plans, performance scores could be published by national accrediting bodies such as the National Committee for Quality Assurance (NCQA). Hospitals could have scores considered by groups such as the Joint Commission on Accreditation of Healthcare Organizations (JCAHO). Publicly available information on quality could potentially inform decisions about care made by consumers and healthcare purchasers.

## ADAPTABILITY

Even though consistency in measurement is often desirable so that trends can be accurately monitored, cancer care data systems need to be flexible so that accommodations can be made for new evidence on quality measures, changes in healthcare delivery, and technological innovation.

## PROTECTIONS TO ENSURE PRIVACY OF
## HEALTH INFORMATION

Maintenance of sensitive personal health information, such as the diagnosis of cancer, in large computerized databases raises serious issues regarding privacy and confidentiality. Legal protections must be in place to ensure that data collection is appropriate, that information is stored securely, and that access to the information is controlled. Federal and state laws and regulations governing privacy, confidentiality, and data security must be strictly enforced while at the same time allowing important registry functions to proceed. Data linkages using personal identifiers such as social security number or birth date, for example, are necessary to eliminate duplicate reports of a case from different healthcare providers. A relatively new application of linkage is the assessment of quality of cancer care.

# 3

# How Are Healthcare Systems
# Monitoring Quality Today?

A wide gulf exits between the ideal data system just described and the reality of cancer care quality monitoring today. Although the United States has no national comprehensive quality monitoring system, there is a patchwork of private and federal efforts to assess cancer care quality. Each initiative operates with different purposes, perspectives, and audiences. Many of the quality (and cost) monitoring activities are organized within hospitals or provider groups, usually in an effort to demonstrate value to the insurers and managed care organizations purchasing their services. Other quality monitoring activities are externally driven and have an accountability function—the government may want to ensure that publicly funded healthcare programs are adhering to best practices, or professional societies may want to demonstrate to the public that their care meets or exceeds accepted standards of care. This chapter first illustrates with a series of case studies the diversity of approaches to cancer care quality monitoring taken by selected individual providers, hospitals, health plans, provider groups, physician practice management companies, insurers, and purchasers. The chapter concludes with a discussion of the strengths and weaknesses of current approaches.

## CASE STUDIES—ILLUSTRATIONS OF THE USE OF
## DATA TO MONITOR CANCER CARE QUALITY

In this section of the report, 10 case studies are presented to show how data are being used within various systems of care to provide information on the quality of cancer care (Table 3.1). The examples range from a single private

**TABLE 3.1** Illustrative Case Studies of Using Cancer Care Data for Quality Monitoring Purposes

| Name (type of organization) | Purpose | Data Source(s) |
|---|---|---|
| 1. Marin Oncology Associates (private oncology practice) | Monitor adherence to guidelines regarding screening, treatment, follow-up, supportive, and end-of-life care | Medical chart |
| 2. OnCare (physician practice management company [PPMC]) | Monitor adherence to guidelines regarding treatment, follow-up, and end-of-life care | Electronic medical chart |
| 3. American College of Radiology | Monitor patterns of care and adherence to treatment guidelines | Medical chart abstraction from a national sample of radiation oncology providers |
| 4. Sutter Health (integrated healthcare delivery system) | Monitor adherence to breast cancer treatment guidelines | Hospital cancer registry, administrative data, medical charts, patient surveys |
| 5. Providence Health Plan (integrated delivery system) | Monitor adherence to breast cancer treatment guidelines | Hospital cancer registry, administrative data, medical charts, patient surveys |
| 6. National Comprehensive Cancer Network (17 large cancer centers) | Monitor adherence to breast cancer treatment guidelines | Medical charts; reporting according to a uniform data set |
| 7. Roswell Park Cancer Institute and private insurers in western New York | Monitor adherence to breast cancer treatment guidelines | Insurance claims, medical charts |
| 8. Colorado Cancer Registry, University of Colorado, and State Medicare Peer Review Organization | Monitor use of adjuvant therapies for breast and colorectal cancer | State cancer registry, Medicare claims, medical charts |
| 9. Central Florida Health Care Coalition (business coalition) | Monitor quality of care for individuals with selected conditions including cancer | Insurance claims, (hospital and outpatient), patient survey |
| 10. National Cancer Data Base (database maintained by the American College of Surgeons and the American Cancer Society) | Monitor quality of care for individuals with cancer | Hospital cancer registries, cancer centers with uniform reporting requirements |

medical office, to large integrated delivery systems, to states. These case studies are not meant to be truly representative of all cancer-related quality improvement programs, but instead were drawn to illustrate the variety of ongoing approaches to using data. The case studies were not identified in any systematic way. Most were identified through contacts with cancer-related health services researchers and IOM workshop participants. Others were identified through descriptions in publications (e.g., the President's Cancer Panel) or presentations at professional meetings (e.g., American Society of Clinical Oncology).

Launching a quality assurance program using only internal resources is unusual for a small group of private practitioners, but Case Study 1 (see box) provides an example of one such initiative. Barriers to quality monitoring identified by members of this small practice included high costs, limited staff resources, a lack of incentives, an absence of an accepted set of quality measures, and a lack of benchmarks or standards with which to gauge success (P. Eisenberg, physician, Marin Oncology Associates, Inc., personal communication, October 18, 1999). According to the practice physicians, the program has been effective in aligning the practice with accepted practice guidelines and in demonstrating the value of the group practice to managed care organizations and insurers (P. Eisenberg, personal communication, October 18, 1999).

Quality assessment is expensive and can usually be accomplished more easily when development costs are spread across groups of providers. Increasingly, provider practice management companies have formed to provide administrative functions for their members, for example, billing and claims processing (Mighion et al., 1999). Case Study 2 is an example of one such company with a unique focus on quality. Its members are small, community-based oncology practices located throughout the country. The program is especially notable because of its use of an electronic medical record system with embedded guidelines, available to providers at the point of contact with patients. Such support systems for clinical decision making can significantly improve the quality of patient care (Classen, 1998; Hunt et al., 1998). Other physician practice management companies and disease management companies are developing electronic medical record systems, and most have a central shared database of clinical, patient, financial, and administrative information.

About one-quarter of OnCare patients have a diagnosis of breast cancer, and, since 1997, OnCare has attempted to standardize the approach to adjuvant treatment to improve outcomes and reduce cost. In general, adherence to the guidelines among OnCare physicians was already good, but giving physicians information on their own performance relative to average practice improved the performance of a few "outlier" physicians. More deviation from guidelines has been found for colon cancer (e.g., overuse of adjuvant therapy for Stage I cancer). In addition to changing practice patterns, the availability of the electronic medical record has improved the recording of stage, comorbid illnesses, medication, prior treatment, and other prognostic indicators (K. Bergstrom, vice president, disease management, OnCare, personal communication, October 26, 1999).

## Case Study 1: Marin Oncology Associates— A Community-Based Private Oncology Practice

Marin Oncology is a San Francisco Bay Area, community-based private practice that has monitored the quality of care provided by its three physicians. The practice has attempted to achieve a patient-centered, evidence-based, and cost-effective practice by establishing standards and a monitoring system. The physicians identified cancer care measures from guidelines, the medical literature, and specialty societies (e.g., American College of Physicians, American Society of Clinical Oncology). Several measures were deemed appropriate to monitor; however, specific benchmarks or targets to gauge success could not be found. The measures finally adopted by the practice address the efficacy of treatment (e.g., survival), processes of care (e.g., use of second-line chemotherapy), and supportive care (e.g., pain management, end-of-life care).

**Breast cancer**
- Proportion of early breast cancer patients receiving mammogram within 12 months of their primary diagnosis.
- American Society of Clinical Oncology Breast cancer follow-up guidelines (e.g., use of routine blood tests, bone scans).

**Non-small-cell lung cancer**
- Proportion of patients with widespread disease (Stage IV) receiving first-, second- and third-line chemotherapy.
- 1- and 2-year survival.

**Chemotherapy**
- Use of second-line chemotherapy for which there is no evidence of therapeutic benefit.
- Use of colony stimulating factors during chemotherapy.

**Pain control**
- Hospitalization rates.

**End-of-life care**
- Hospice use, length of stay.
- Site of death (home, hospital, Extended Care Facility).
- Interval from last chemotherapy to death.
- Use of form documenting patient preferences for care (e.g., advanced directives, do not resuscitate orders).

Data are retrieved through chart audit and are summarized on Excel spreadsheets. Much of the work is done by the clinicians and their staff, but some analytic support has come from Public Health residents from Loma Linda University.

SOURCE: P. Eisenberg, physician, Marin Oncology Associates, Inc., personal communication, October 18, 1999.

---

### Case Study 2:  OnCare—A Physician Practice Management Company

OnCare is a privately held, for-profit, physician practice management company with a focus on guideline-driven quality improvement. The company owns and manages medical and radiation oncology offices and clinics in 11 states. The 28 physician practices that are affiliated with OnCare have replaced paper medical records with an electronic charting system that includes embedded on-line decision support for all aspects of care (e.g., choice of initial therapy, dosage of chemotherapy, supportive care). Information about patient care is captured, analyzed, and fed back to the system's more than 100 physicians to assess their compliance to the guidelines. To date, the system includes information on more than 15,000 patients.

OnCare clinicians enter patient data in a flow chart format as the patient is receiving care. Clinical options are displayed allowing providers to consider guideline recommendations as decisions about care are being made (e.g., selection of chemotherapy). Furthermore, providers can examine the processes of care and outcomes of patients within the OnCare system who have characteristics similar to the patient being evaluated. The OnCare electronic medical chart is called KnowChart® and was developed by a software vendor, KnowMed Systems. The electronic medical record is integrated with laboratory systems, patient scheduling, and billing.

OnCare guidelines have been developed for most cancer sites/types and are integrated into the information system. The guidelines were developed according to a review of the literature, advice of experts, and input from local OnCare providers. If providers wish to deviate from the guidelines, they must document their rationale for doing so. Reasons for changing chemotherapy doses are also documented in the system.

OnCare provides its practices with information on clinical and financial performance, as well as marketing support. OnCare is expanding. It has, for example, entered into a partnership with the not-for-profit M.D. Anderson Cancer Network to develop and market a managed-care plan

SOURCES: G. Swanson, physician, OnCare, personal communication, October 26, 1999; K. Bergstrom, vice president, disease management, OnCare, personal communication, October 26, 1999; R. Shiffman, physician, OnCare, personal communication, October 26, 1999; www.oncare.com; www.know med.com.

---

Adherence to other cancer care guidelines has also been assessed using OnCare's clinical information system. In 1996, for example, OnCare providers assessed their compliance to the 1994 American Society of Clinical Oncology's guidelines on the use of hematopoietic growth factors. Information relevant to end-of-life care is being tracked to assess the success of a physician training program in end-of-life care (K. Bergstrom, vice president, disease management, OnCare, personal communication, October 26, 1999).

Case Study 3 provides another example of the centralization of quality improvement activities for a particular group of providers. The American College

## Case Study 3:  Quality Monitoring of Radiation Oncology Care, American College of Radiology

ACR has, since 1973, monitored the quality of U.S. radiation oncology care with support from NCI. ACR's "Patterns of Care Study" (PCS) process begins with the development of a consensus guideline that summarizes what is determined to be the "best current management" for a particular cancer. Panels are convened to review available evidence and develop decision trees for patient management. In developing the guideline, panelists may assess treatment modality, type of equipment, dose ranges, and treatment areas for radiation therapy. If there is disagreement among the panel members, a formal process is used to reach consensus (i.e., modified Delphi process). Panels also develop questions for a national survey of providers to assess how care is actually being delivered to patients and whether there is deviation from the guidelines.

The next step of the PCS process is obtaining data on processes of care, and sometimes outcomes of care through a nationwide survey of radiation oncology providers. Independent surveyors visit selected radiation facilities, abstract information from a sample of their medical charts, and enter the data into laptop computers. Typically, 75 facilities and 10 cases per facility are represented for each cancer-specific study. Information on outcomes may be collected at the same time that processes of care data are gathered, or in the case of 5-year survival, years following the original survey. ACR staff researchers aggregate and analyze the survey data to ascertain patterns of care, the consistency of practice to guidelines, and the nature of interactions of structures of care, processes of care, and outcomes.

The ability to generalize survey findings to the nation is possible because samples of radiation oncology providers are carefully drawn from a comprehensive list of facilities maintained by ACR. All radiation oncology departments in the United States are included in the listing, along with information about resources at each site (e.g., size, equipment, personnel). For the PCS survey, a sample of facilities is selected to ensure that all sizes and types of facilities are appropriately represented; then a sample of patients from each of these facilities is randomly selected from those eligible for the study. This process minimizes bias that could occur if facilities were to select their own cases for inclusion. Sometimes, certain facilities are sampled at higher rates so that statistically valid subgroup comparisons can be made (e.g., for studies of care of minority populations).

A total of 29 PCS studies have been conducted to date (see Table 3.2), providing insights into the quality of U.S. radiation oncology care.

SOURCES: J. Owen, director, Patterns of Care Study, American College of Radiology, personal communication, November 12, 1999; Coia LR, Owen JB, Hanks GE, 1997, "Introduction" *Seminars in Radiation Oncology* 7(2):95–96; Hanks GE, Coia LR, Curry J, 1997, "Patterns of Care Studies: Past, Present, and Future," *Seminars in Radiation Oncology* 7(2):97–100.

**TABLE 3.2**  Patterns of Care Studies, 1973–1999

| Disease Site | Years of Treatment |
|---|---|
| Cervix | 1973, 1978, 1983, 1988–1989, 1992–1994 |
| Prostate | 1973–1975, 1978, 1983, 1989, 1994 |
| Hodgkin's disease | 1973, 1983, 1988–1989 |
| Breast | 1973, 1983, 1989, 1993–1994 |
| Larynx | 1973–1975, 1978 |
| Bladder | 1973–1975 |
| Corpus uteri | 1973 |
| Nasopharynx | 1973–1975 |
| Testicular seminoma | 1973, 1992–1994 |
| Tongue | 1973–1975 |
| Palliation | 1983 |
| Rectum | 1988–1989, 1992–1994 |
| Esophagus | 1992–1994 |
| Tonsil | 1976–1985 |

SOURCE: J. Owen, director, Patterns of Care Study, American College of Radiology, personal communication, November 12, 1999.

of Radiology (ACR) has developed a system to monitor the quality of radiation oncology care throughout the United States. Since 1973, ACR has identified best practices through guideline development, then conducted extensive targeted surveys of practitioners to evaluate adherence to the guidelines. The ACR effort is laudable because of its adherence to good sampling and data collection techniques, allowing it to provide accurate information on the quality of radiation oncology care for the nation. The program was not designed to provide information about quality to individual practices or institutions. Instead, quality improvement is promoted through ACR's educational activities (e.g., dissemination of patterns of care information in journals and professional meetings) and standards and practice accreditation programs. The program has long-standing financial support from the National Cancer Institute (NCI). In 1999, ACR received over $700,000 to support their quality program (F. Mahoney, Grants Office, NCI, personal communication, November 30, 1999).

Quality systems described thus far have been limited to the care of certain providers, either oncologists or radiation oncologists. Cancer care is multidisciplinary and, within larger systems of care, quality improvement programs need to address the range of services needed by individuals with cancer. Case Study 4 illustrates how such cross-cutting quality measures can be applied within a large integrated system of hospitals and medical groups. Sutter Health has developed a quality improvement program for breast cancer and has put in place an information system to record compliance to quality algorithms. Sources of quality information include the hospital cancer registry, administrative and clinical records, and patient surveys. With 2 years of data collected thus far, there is some evidence of success—there has been improvement for six of the eight measures. Significant variation remains, however, among the system's hospitals and medical groups (Katterhagen, 1999).

Case Study 5 illustrates how Providence Health System, a large integrated delivery system, has adopted measures originally developed by the Foundation

---

### Case Study 4:  Sutter Health Breast Cancer Quality Project

Sutter Health is an integrated system of 23 acute care hospitals and 8 allied medical groups in Northern California. Since 1997, Sutter Health has monitored the quality and costs of breast cancer care throughout its system to improve clinical outcomes, reduce costs, and increase market share for hospitals, medical groups, and physicians. The quality monitoring system was initially developed in 1994 in selected facilities within the system (i.e., the Mills-Peninsula Health Services).

Data from the hospital cancer registry, State cancer registry, hospital administrative systems, breast center clinical systems, and patient surveys are used to track the following measures (targets are for 1999):

• size or stage at diagnosis (with appropriate levels of screening, should see early stage disease, for example, ductal carcinoma in situ [DCIS] rate should exceed 21%);
• needle biopsy rates (should be high relative to surgical biopsy, exceeding 50%);
• axillary dissection rates for DCIS (should be 2% or lower);
• surgical breast conservation rates (should exceed 65% for early stage disease);
• radiation therapy as a component of surgical conservation (should exceed 85%, but be reduced for selected patient groups);
• adjuvant chemotherapy for Stage II, node positive cases (should exceed 95%);
• patient satisfaction (no targets established); and
• patient quality of life (use the Functional Assessment of Cancer Therapy-Breast quality-of-life instrument [FACT-B]) (no targets established).

The performance of individual hospitals and medical groups relative to practice algorithms is reported by name on a quarterly basis, along with group norms and targets, and is disseminated at tumor board and departmental meetings, via newsletters, and for "outliers" on an individual basis. Local senior management and medical directors are held accountable for performance.

SOURCE: G. Katterhagen, personal communication, October 4, 1999.

for Accountability (FACCT) for breast cancer. These measures are quite comprehensive and include indicators of the processes of care, patient satisfaction, and outcomes (Table 3.3).

The case studies described so far have relied almost exclusively on clinical data recorded in the chart, data available from the hospital cancer registry, and hospital administrative records. Case Study 6 illustrates an alternative mechanism, the development of a very expensive clinical information system. Seventeen of the nation's premier cancer centers have joined together to form the National Comprehensive Cancer Network (NCCN) in an effort to measure and monitor the quality of care within the member institutions (Figure 3.1).

In collaboration with one of the NCCN member institutions, Roswell Park Cancer Institute, a coalition of managed care organizations and insurers has banded together to assess the quality of care for the entire insured population of western New York State. This effort is described in Case Study 7. From a data perspective, the approach taken is quite unique. Cases are first identified through insurance claims; then medical records are abstracted to obtain information on stage of illness. Analyses of the supplemented claims data provide information on the quality of breast cancer care.

---

**Case Study 5:  Providence Health System**

Providence Health System is an integrated delivery system with over 50 medical centers in Oregon, Washington, and Alaska. Since 1993, the Providence Health Plan of Oregon has monitored several clinical measures on all breast cancer patients diagnosed and/or treated in the health system: stage at diagnosis, rate of breast-conserving surgery (BCS), radiation treatment after BCS, chemotherapy for node positive disease, Tamoxifen for ER positive disease, and overall survival. These clinical measures are derived from reports from the hospital cancer registry reporting system and the medical chart. A sample of patients is contacted by mail to complete a survey regarding their satisfaction and experience with care.

Providers within the system are apprised of the results of monitoring through an annual cancer program report, cancer committee meetings, tumor boards, and various regional quality improvement teams. No attempt has been made to give providers information on their individual performance. Since 1993 there have been increases in the share of patients diagnosed with early stage disease, the rate of BCS for early stage disease (from about 33 to 60% from 1993 to 1999), and use of radiation following surgery (from 76 to 84% from 1994 to 1998). The chemotherapy and tamoxifen measures were just introduced in 1999, and there are as yet insufficient data to report.

SOURCE: L. Skokan, senior scientist, Providence Health System, personal communication, November 23, 1999.

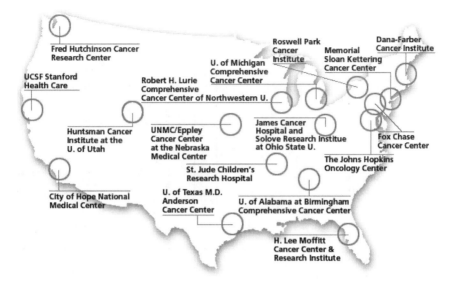

**FIGURE 3.1** National Comprehensive Cancer Network member institutions. SOURCE: National Comprehensive Cancer Network. 1999. Member Institutions. http://www.nccn. org/network_content.htm.

None of the case studies described thus far have provided quality-of-care information for all cancer patients residing within a specific geographic area. Case Study 8 comes close to achieving this by providing information on some aspects of the quality of breast and colon cancer care for the elderly residents of Colorado. This case study illustrates the potential for collaborative efforts involving cancer registries, universities, and Peer Review Organizations (PROs) to improve cancer care quality. Each state has a PRO funded by the Health Care Financing Administration (HCFA). The PROs evaluate whether care given to Medicare patients is reasonable, necessary, and provided in the most appropriate setting. The most recent contract with HCFA requires the PROs to conduct local quality improvement projects focused on six clinical prioritized areas, one of them breast cancer (Jencks, 1999).

Case Study 9 provides an example of employers joining together to form a large coalition to push for uniform quality assessment among the health plans covering their employees. Purchasers may use quality information to identify high-value plans, to steer employees into higher-performing plans, or as leverage when establishing rates for premiums (Darby, 1998).

The last case study represents perhaps the largest single effort to monitor cancer care in the United States. The National Cancer Data Base (NCDB) includes quality-related information on more than three-quarters of newly diagnosed cases of cancer. The effort is jointly sponsored by the American College of Surgeons' Commission on Cancer (ACoS-CoC) and the American Cancer Society.

**TABLE 3.3** Foundation for Accountability (FACCT) Breast Cancer Quality Indicators

| Measure | Performance Value | Instrument or Data Source |
| --- | --- | --- |
| **Steps to Good Care** | | |
| Mammography | Proportion of women age 52–69 who have had a mammogram within 2 years | Doctor's billing or claims records (NCQA's HEDIS® 3.0 breast cancer screening measure used) |
| Early-stage detection | Proportion of patients whose breast cancer was detected at Stage 0 or Stage I | Patient records from cancer registry |
| Information about radiation treatment options | Proportion of Stage I and II patients who indicate that they had adequate information about their radiation treatment options before deciding about treatment | One question in patient satisfaction survey completed 3–6 months after diagnosis |
| Breast conserving surgery (BCS) | Proportion of Stage I and II patients who undergo BCS | Patient records from cancer registry or claims records |
| Radiation therapy following BCS | Proportion of BCS patients who receive radiation treatment after surgery | Patient records from cancer registry or claims records |

**Experience and Satisfaction**

Patient satisfaction with care — Mean score for patients' level of satisfaction with breast cancer care, including the technical quality, interpersonal and communication skills of their cancer doctor, their involvement in treatment decisions, and the timeliness of receiving information and services — 32-item patient satisfaction survey completed 3–6 months after diagnosis

**Results**

Experience of disease — Mean score for patients on CARES-SF survey, which assesses patients' quality of life and experience in living with breast cancer — 59-item CARES-SF patient survey completed 12–15 months after diagnosis

5-year disease-free survival (cancer treatment center measure) — Probability of disease-free survival for a group of patients, Stages I–IV, who were diagnosed during previous 5 years — Patient records from cancer registry

NOTE: CARES = Cancer Rehabilitation Evaluation System.

SOURCE: Foundation for Accountability, 1998. FACCT Quality Measures—Breast Cancer. Available on line at: http://www.facct.org.

---

**Case Study 6:  The National Comprehensive Cancer Network**

NCCN institutions cooperated to develop a set of clinical practice guide-lines for the treatment of common cancers. Available sources of data were determined to be inadequate to monitor adherence to the guidelines, and an extensive uniform clinical data set was defined to guide data collection. Now detailed sociodemographic, clinical, treatment, outcome, and cost data are gathered on all patients with selected cancers treated in the NCCN network. Data are used to evaluate both the performance of providers relative to the guidelines and the effectiveness of treatments. The database is very exten-sive; for breast cancer alone, over 200 data elements are collected.

Data managers from each cancer center report encrypted data via the internet to a central analytic office. Strict data security and confidentiality measures are in place (e.g., individual authentication of users, stripping per-sonal identifiers from records), as are methods to ensure the quality of data (e.g., standardized coding schemes, audits). Performance results are posted on a Web page accessible to providers within the system.

Data collection for the pilot condition—breast cancer—began in July 1997. As of October 1999, information on over 2,000 patients had been entered into the system. Preliminary results show high compliance to guidelines but some areas of practice variation. Among women treated with BCS, for example, 89% received radiation therapy overall, with a range across institutions from 80 to 100%.

Plans are to expand to other cancer sites and to add information on com-plications and patient-reported quality of life. The NCCN would like to extend participation to selected outside institutions/practices and to establish new partnerships with pharmaceutical and biotechnology companies, insurers, and regulatory/accrediting bodies.

SOURCE: Weeks, 1999.

---

ACoS-CoC regularly conducts surveys of facilities that provide cancer treatment and approves those that meet its standards.[*] Approximately 1,500 pro-grams have been approved, which are estimated to provide care for 80% of the nation's newly diagnosed patients (Morrow, 1999). Most facilities are commu-nity-based hospitals, but a few freestanding cancer programs are also included (Table 3.4) (Morrow, 1999).

---

[*]The Joint Commission on Accreditation of Healthcare Organizations as of January 1999 accepts the American College of Surgeons' Commission on Cancer accreditation decisions for cancer treatment facilities or cancer hospitals that are affiliated with health plans and health systems (www.facs.org). This will effectively reduce the redundancy of site evaluations of cancer facilities.

## Case Study 7:  Implementing a Regional Cancer Quality Monitoring Program Using Private Insurance Claims Data

A regional total quality management program for cancer care is being developed in western New York State through a collaboration of the Roswell Park Cancer Institute, the Independent Health Association (IHA), a managed care organization, and a board of community physicians. The first phase of the project involved a retrospective quality review of breast cancer care in 1995 and 1996. Under development is the second phase, a prospective quality improvement program that will involve interventions such as:

- reporting of aggregate and provider-specific data to specialty physicians,
- distributing guidelines and aggregate data to primary providers,
- case management through payers, and
- disseminating treatment guidelines to the public.

As part of phase I, IHA's breast cancer-related claims from 1995 to 1996 were analyzed to assess compliance to guidelines of the NCCN. Claims that included ICD-9 diagnostic and CPT procedure codes indicative of a diagnosis of breast cancer were collected into a Microsoft Access database. For patients whose sequence of procedures and other care was consistent with a diagnosis of breast cancer, medical records (pathology and operative reports) were retrieved by IHA to confirm the diagnosis and to determine the cancer stage. Case identification generally occurs 6 to 9 months after diagnosis allowing for timely quality evaluation. Virtually all cancer cases were identified using claims data according to results of a validation study.

Quality indicators included:

**Diagnosis**
- Positive rate for mammographic directed breast biopsy.
- Use of needle biopsy for diagnosis.

**Work-up**
- Rate of use of bone scan, computerized tomography, and serum tumor markers.

**Surgery**
- Rate of reexcision by biopsy type with breast conserving surgery (BCS).
- Rate of BCS.
- Rate of immediate breast reconstruction.

**Guideline Compliance**
- Rate of variation from NCCN guidelines for surgery, radiation, and adjuvant systemic therapy.

*Continued*

**Case Study 7:** *Continued*

The study demonstrated a rate of BCS higher than the national average and overall high rates of compliance with NCCN guidelines. Provider-specific data analysis showed substantial variation between physicians in the use of biopsy techniques and the rate of positive biopsies. Treatment-related quality problems identified among the 379 women with Stage 0/I/II breast cancer identified in 1995–1996 included:

- 13% of women (5 of 38 women) with DCIS treated with BCS had axillary lymph node dissection (not indicated with DCIS),
- 10% of women (18 of 188 women) did not receive radiation therapy following breast conserving therapy when this was indicated,
- 8% of women (8 of 105 women) were treated with radiation therapy following mastectomy when the treatment was not indicated (i.e., they had fewer than 4 positive nodes and tumors less than 5 cm), and
- 68% of women (19 of 28 women) were not treated with radiation therapy following mastectomy when the treatment was indicated (i.e., they had 4 or more positive nodes).

Designers of this program estimate that the initial data collection and analysis of claims data for breast cancer among an insured population of 1 million can be accomplished with a relatively small budget (under $150,000).

Plans are to extend the program to monitor the quality of other common cancers (i.e., colon, lung, prostate, lymphoma). The current program covers an estimated 25% of the population in the region, but with the anticipated cooperation of other insurers (e.g., Blue Cross Blue Shield of western New York and Univera), a comprehensive quality assurance program could reach up to 90% of the insured population of western New York. The program will also define mechanisms to include nonmanaged Medicare and uninsured patients.

SOURCE: S. B. Edge, chief, Breast Department, Division of Surgical Oncology, Roswell Park Cancer Institute, personal communication, November 3, 1999.

**Case Study 8: Monitoring the Quality of Breast and Colon Cancer Treatment Among Medicare Beneficiaries in Colorado**

The quality of cancer care for Medicare beneficiaries in Colorado was assessed through a collaborative effort of the University of Colorado Cancer Center, the Colorado Central Cancer Registry, and the Colorado Foundation for Medical Care (the state Peer Review Organization responsible for Medicare quality initiatives funded by the Health Care Financing Administration). Data from the state's central cancer registry were linked to Medicare administrative records (parts A and B claims) to assess the appropriate use of: (1) adjuvant radiotherapy following lumpectomy for women with Stage I and II breast cancer and (2) adjuvant chemotherapy following surgery for people with

Stage III colon cancer. These therapies have been proven to improve 5-year outcomes (i.e., reduce local recurrence, increase survival) and are appropriate for individuals with a life expectancy of at least 5 years. Life expectancy in Colorado is more than 10 years for those having reached age 75, and so underuse of adjuvant therapies among the elderly can serve as a population-based indicator of poor care.

Cancer registry data for patients diagnosed in 1994 and 1995 with breast or colon cancer were matched with the Medicare master beneficiary file for Colorado. After matching, information from the Medicare Part A inpatient billing file and the Medicare Part B outpatient billing file was added to the analytic file. Thereafter, all personal identifiers were removed from the data set. Analyses were conducted on a statewide basis, without regard to the specific identities of either the communities, healthcare providers, or hospitals. During the study period, roughly one-quarter of Medicare beneficiaries were enrolled in HMOs. HMOs do not submit diagnosis and treatment data to Medicare; therefore, information on use of adjuvant therapies among HMO members was limited to data from the cancer registry. The registry captured information on radiotherapy quite well, but it missed a sizable share of chemotherapy treatments. The medical charts of patients who did not receive adjuvant therapies were reviewed to verify that they had not been used (83% of records were obtained for review).

Only 72% of women aged 65 and older received adjuvant radiotherapy following lumpectomy for Stage I and II breast cancer, and only 52% of individuals treated surgically for Stage III colon cancer received adjuvant chemotherapy. Investigators assessed the role of a number of factors potentially associated with underuse of adjuvant therapy, including age, gender, race, place of residence (metro vs. nonmetro area), type of medical insurance (fee-for-service vs. HMO), tumor size and grade, and comorbidity (as captured from Medicare Part A hospital records). The principal determinant of use of adjuvant therapies was age. The increasing prevalence of comorbidities with advancing age had a minimal role in the less frequent use of adjuvant therapy after age 65. Reviews of medical charts indicated that patient refusal was rarely the reason therapies were not used.

To disseminate the study findings and improve care, a short (17 minute) video was made and distributed to hospital tumor boards and registrars around the state, findings were published in a newsletter mailed to all physicians in the state, and presentations were given at professional conferences. Response on the part of providers has been generally positive. To better understand why adjuvant therapies are being underused among the elderly in Colorado, a new study has been launched of physician–patient interactions in decision-making about adjuvant chemotherapy for colorectal cancer. The Medicare-registry matching study will be redone in 2000 on cases diagnosed from 1996 to 1998 to assess progress.

SOURCE: T. Byers, principal investigator, University of Colorado Cancer Center, personal communication, October 7, 1999.

---

**Case Study 9:  Central Florida Health Care Coalition**

The Central Florida Health Care Coalition (CFHCC) represents area businesses, including Walt Disney World, Universal Studios, Lockheed Martin, as well as public employers, that together insure nearly 900,000 individuals. Employees of coalition members are covered by eight health insurance plans. CFHCC has for 8 years used Atlas® data to monitor inpatient care. Patient satisfaction with care is assessed using the Consumer Assessment of Health Plans Survey (CAHPS), developed by the Agency for Healthcare Research and Quality. CFHCC has analyzed data from the state cancer registry regarding breast cancer treatment, but difficulties with data from cancer registries, such as inaccurate information on stage of diagnosis, led the coalition to pool other sources of data to assess cancer care quality. CFHCC has recently turned its attention to the quality of outpatient care and has contracted with a private firm, ProtoCare Sciences, to develop an extensive claims database that will include claims for outpatient care for three of the Coalition employers. Attention will initially be focused on 10 noncancer diagnosis-related groups (DRGs) (e.g., cholesterol control, depression) and 5 physician groups (i.e., family practice, internal medicine, gastroenterology, cardiology, obstetrics-gynecology). Profiles of care will be developed for each physician with a case load of at least 30 for the given indication. Plans are to expand the database to include other conditions such as breast cancer and to profile cancer care providers such as surgeons and oncologists.

SOURCE: Becky J. Cherney, President/CEO, CFHCC, personal communication, November 23, 1999.

---

## SUMMARY

As the case studies illustrate, available data resources provide a number of ways to implement quality improvement programs. Some programs depend entirely on retrospective reviews of medical charts or hospital cancer registries while others rely on multiple sources, for example, administrative claims data linked to cancer registry data. The case studies are, in fact, a testament to creativity—data intended for other purposes have in several instances been manipulated to monitor quality care, and sometimes appear to have been used within programs to effect improvements in care.

The case studies demonstrate several barriers to systematic quality monitoring. First, because of a lack of recognized measures of quality, provider groups or organizations have themselves frequently assumed the task of reviewing evidence, developing guidelines, and identifying measures. These activities are very costly undertakings, require considerable expertise, and need to be continually reviewed in light of new evidence. Many of the systems could have benefited from an established set of quality measures. The development of

**TABLE 3.4** Facilities Approved by American College of Surgeons' Commission on Cancer, 1999

| Category | No. | Percent |
|---|---|---|
| Total | 1,479 | 100% |
| Community Hospital Cancer Program | 631 | 3 |
| Community Hospital Comprehensive Program (>300 analytic cases/year) | 465 | 31 |
| Teaching Hospital Cancer Program | 314 | 21 |
| NCI-designated programs | 23 | 2 |
| All others (e.g., freestanding cancer program offering two of three treatment modalities; single modality centers) | 46 | 3 |

SOURCE: Morrow, 1999.

---

**Case Study 10: The National Cancer Data Base**

A major initiative of the Commission on Cancer, in collaboration with the American Cancer Society, is NCDB, which collects data from 1,600 hospitals and other facilities in all 50 states. Since 1996, all approved facilities have been required to report all of their cases for 38 cancer sites to the program. Data are also collected from facilities that are not approved. In 1997, 835,000 cases were reported to NCDB. Each participating hospital is given back its own data in summary form, which it can use to compare with national data. The national data allow problem areas to be pinpointed (e.g., widespread use of an inappropriate treatment for a particular type of cancer) and trends to be observed over time in such characteristics as stage at diagnosis, percentage of patients who have complete staging information, and type of treatment given. Results of NCDB analyses are published regularly in professional journals (Bland et al., 1998; Sener et al., 1999).

In addition to routine data collection, each year two Patient Care Evaluation (PCE) studies are carried out, focusing on specific cancer types or general treatment issues. Since 1977, 33 PCE studies have been conducted. Recent PCE studies have focused on colorectal cancer and Non-Hodgkin's lymphoma. More extensive data are collected for these special studies, allowing a more detailed analysis of how patients are treated, with the data again fed back to hospitals for comparison in the national spectrum.

SOURCE: Morrow, 1999.

---

guidelines through NCCN seems to have spurred quality monitoring activities beyond the cancer centers that developed them (e.g., the Roswell Park Cancer Institute initiative), and the development of breast cancer quality indicators by FACCT seems to have also promoted measurement activities (e.g., Providence

Health System). If an available set of core cancer care measures were available, it would likely be adopted.

Likewise, virtually no benchmarks exist with which to gauge success. Systems sometimes establish internal benchmarks based on practice norms, but they often have no way to know whether their performance is better or worse than that of providers outside their practice system. In addition, some statistical issues, if not taken into account, may skew benchmarks (e.g., providers with small numbers of cases unduly affecting norms).

Again, these case studies may not represent well the scope of quality assessment activities in cancer care, but they would suggest that relatively little attention is being paid to the full spectrum of cancer care, for example, the quality of pain management and end-of-life care.

# 4

# The Data Infrastructure for
# Health Services Research

This chapter describes data resources for cancer-related health services re-search, the study of the structure, processes, and effects of healthcare services. Relative to funding for basic cancer research, support for research in this field is quite modest (IOM, 1999a). Even so, the agencies supporting health services research and investigators in this field have developed innovative methods to enhance available data resources through linkages, special studies, the establishment of research consortiums, and new data collection initiatives. This chapter begins with a description of selected programs that take advantage of current data systems to further cancer-related health services research, and concludes with a discussion of the limitations of federally funded surveys when applied to quality-of-care issues.

## LINKAGE OF CANCER REGISTRIES TO
## ADMINISTRATIVE DATA

A great deal has been learned about the quality of cancer care from studies that link two or more complementary data sources. The linkage of cancer registry data to insurance claims databases, for example, has provided evidence of significant geographic variations in care and has suggested that care within certain HMOs for certain cancers is as good as, or superior to, the care provided in fee-for-service plans (Potosky et al., 1997; Riley et al., 1999).

Registry data contain useful measures of severity of cancer (e.g., cancer stage) and date of diagnosis but may lack complete information on treatment and outcomes. Claims-based data may lack certain diagnostic information but include detailed information on the cost and use of medical services (Fleming and Kohrs, 1998). Claims data are often accessible, routinely collected, and represent the utilization experience of a large number of patients. Their limitations, however, include coding misspecification and errors, incomplete listing of extant disease (e.g., listing only a limited number of diagnoses on hospital discharge files), and difficulties in distinguishing incident from prevalent conditions (e.g., whether a condition listed arose during a hospitalization or was preexisting).

One of the most fruitful linkages for cancer care assessment is that of the Surveillance, Epidemiology, and End Results (SEER) cancer registries to claims records in Medicare's administrative database (Moulton, 1998). This is a collaborative effort of the National Cancer Institute (NCI), the SEER registries, and the Health Care Financing Administration (HCFA) to create a large population-based source of information for cancer-related epidemiologic and health services research (Potosky et al., 1993). The SEER registries are located in 11 geographic areas and 3 supplemental registries that include 14% of the U.S. population (SEER registries are described more fully in Chapter 5). The Medicare utilization data (claims) cover stays in institutions (i.e., hospitals and skilled nursing facilities), physician and lab services, hospital outpatient visits, and home health and hospice use. Information on noncovered services such as prescription drugs, and long-term care is not included. The currently available linked file includes all Medicare data through 1998 for persons diagnosed with cancer in 1996.

Matching a case from the cancer registry to claims in the Medicare files is performed using a computer program that applies an algorithm to determine whether records from the two sources represent the same individual based on available identifying information (i.e., social security number, name, birth date, gender). Of persons age 65 and older reported by the SEER registries, 93% were matched to the Medicare master enrollment files. A failure to match may occur if the patient identified in the registry is not a Medicare beneficiary (e.g., an estimated 3% of the elderly do not qualify for Medicare) or errors are made in recording identifying information.

Once a match is established, Medicare claims are extracted. The database includes claims for beneficiaries receiving fee-for-service care and excludes information about care provided to individuals cared for in HMOs, those in the Department of Veterans Affairs (VA) medical system, and those whose care is paid for exclusively with private health insurance. Before release, all information that can identify an individual is stripped from the files. Data files are made available for research on a limited basis through an application process. Representatives from NCI, the SEER registries, and HCFA review each proposal to ensure that the research does not compromise the confidentiality of patients or medical care providers in SEER areas. Researchers who use the SEER-Medicare files must sign agreements to abide by strict confidentiality rules.

The SEER–Medicare data offer an opportunity to examine patterns of care prior to the diagnosis of cancer, during the period of initial diagnosis, and during long-term follow-up. Topics that can be addressed with the linked database include patterns of care for specific cancers, the use of health services, and the costs of treatment (Deleyiannis et al., 1997; Du et al., 1999; Lu-Yao et al., 1996; Potosky et al., 1999; Riley et al., 1999). Longitudinal surveillance of the health care of persons with cancer is another potential use of this linked file. These data can be used to assess health care directed toward the prevention of disease or disability, as well as the restoration or maintenance of health (Edwards, 1997). A control sample of individuals who do not have cancer is available so that comparisons can be made, for example, on healthcare costs for individuals with and without cancer (NCI/SIG, 1999; Warren et al., 1999). Active projects using the linked SEER–Medicare database include analyses of:

- total lifetime payments for elderly cancer patients,
- differences in patterns of care and cancer survival between HMOs and fee-for-service providers,
- breast cancer treatment patterns and trends,
- prostate cancer detection practices,
- trends and variations in initial treatment for early-stage prostate cancer, and
- hospice use among beneficiaries with colorectal and lung cancer.

State cancer registry data have also been linked to Medicare claims (Hillner, 1995; Smith et al., 1995), private insurance claims (Hillner, 1997), and hospital discharge data (Ayanian et al., 1993; Polednak et al., 1996) to assess quality of care (see a listing of selected state registry-based quality studies in Appendix C). The inclusion of the social security number on reports to the National Program of Cancer Registries (NPCR) state registries facilitates successful linkages.

One study under way will test the use of multiple data linkages to assess the quality of cancer care (Box 4.1). If successful, it could foster public reporting of risk-adjusted quality measures for health plans or providers, provide techniques to develop benchmarking standards for internal quality improvement, and establish a standard for surveys of patients' appraisals of care.

## CANCER REGISTRIES AS A SAMPLING FRAME FOR SPECIAL STUDIES

Another mechanism used to assess quality of care is to use cancer registries as a sampling frame for special studies. The registries often have near complete ascertainment of incident cases of cancer but lack additional information needed for quality studies (e.g., information on outpatient treatments). Data elements needed to answer specific questions can be obtained through medical chart abstraction and/or patient survey from a representative sample of cases.

NCI has, since 1988, conducted a series of patterns-of-care studies using this model. NCI's intent is to describe the dissemination of state-of-the-art can cer treatment and explanatory factors for variations in patterns of care. Currently, data are being collected on cases diagnosed in 1998 within SEER registries with cancer of the prostate, corpus uteri, pancreas, and chronic lymphocytic

---

**BOX 4.1  Using State Cancer Registries Linked to Other Data to Assess the Quality of Cancer Care**

An ambitious study under way in California is attempting to capitalize on the strengths of State cancer registry data while compensating for their weaknesses. Investigators at the Harvard Medical School are collaborating with the California Cancer Registry to assess the following process and outcome measures for individuals with colorectal cancer:

- stage at diagnosis,
- timeliness of treatment,
- provision of recommended chemotherapy and radiation therapy,
- patient reported quality of care, and
- survival.

As a first step, the investigators will contact all the physicians who cared for patients with colorectal cancer that were reported to the registry in 1996–1997. Information reported to the cancer registry will be verified and some additional information about the patient's care will be collected, for example, the types of drugs used and the timing of treatment. If the registry data is found to be inaccurate, they will assess whether certain types of hospitals or areas are prone to poor reporting.

Next, the cancer registry data will be linked to a number of data files:

| Type of File | Information Provided |
|---|---|
| Medicare enrollment data (beneficiaries age 65 and older) | Type of health plan and the name of the plan—most people with colorectal cancer are elderly |
| Hospital discharge abstracts | Comorbid conditions identified at the time of surgery |
| Physician specialty data | Training of the physician who reported the cancer |
| U.S. Census data | The patient's area of residence, for example, the level of poverty in the neighborhood |

When all of the files are linked, the investigators will have a fairly comprehensive database with which to evaluate the correlates of good care, for example, whether care was received in a managed care vs. a fee-for-service system, and the type of physician providing care. To gain the patients' perspective on care, the investigators plan to interview a sample of patients 6 months after their diagnosis was made regarding their experience with care (e.g., coordination and continuity of care, physical comfort, trust in doctors and health plans). Aspects of the patients' quality of life will also be assessed, for example, their functional and emotional well-being.

SOURCE: Ayanian, 1999.

leukemia.[1] Participating cancer registries reabstract hospital records for additional data and verify data regarding therapies with physicians. An NCI patterns-of-care study typically takes 5 years from conception to publication of results.

Sampling from SEER registries is also central to NCI's special studies, a mechanism to collect in-depth data beyond that routinely collected for cancer registration (NCI/SIG, 1999). With a time frame of 1 to 2 years, these studies can provide a rapid response to questions of national importance. A SEER study, for example, was used to obtain improved estimates of the risks associated with tamoxifen during a controversial period of the Primary Prevention Trial of Breast Cancer. One of the larger special studies, the Prostate Cancer Outcomes Study, is addressing health-related quality-of-life issues among the increasing population of men identified with prostate cancer who have had radical prostactectomy. As part of this study, a cohort of 3,500 men with prostate cancer was identified from six SEER registries, and health-related quality of life is being measured at 6, 12, and 24 months and at 5 years following diagnosis. Community practice patterns are also being assessed, for example, variations in diagnostic and treatment interventions. The experience with the prostate cancer special study indicates that incident case cohorts can be successfully identified and tracked longitudinally using an existing data collection infrastructure (i.e., the SEER cancer registries) (Potosky, 1999; Potosky et al., 1999).

The American Cancer Society (ACS) is sampling cases from a few state cancer registries as part of a pilot test for two large population-based surveys of cancer survivors (Baker, 1999). The first is a planned 10-year prospective study of survivors enrolled within the first year after diagnosis of any one of the 10

---

[1]Samples of cases from SEER were obtained in 1988, 1989, 1990, 1991, 1995, and 1996 to assess the following cancers: in situ and early-stage breast cancer, colorectal, ovarian, urinary bladder, melanoma, non-small-cell lung, head and neck, cervix, childhood brain stem, and other childhood cancers.

most common cancers.[2] The major aim of the survey is to examine the behavioral, psychosocial, treatment, and support factors that influence quality of life and survival of cancer patients. Plans are to extend the study to other states that have adequate cancer registration and an interest in participating, with the ultimate goal of enrolling a sufficient number of subjects to provide state-level estimates (i.e., up to 100,000 subjects nationwide). Difficulties encountered during the pilot phase of the study have included:

- the lack of rapid case ascertainment mechanisms to identify cases early enough to administer a survey within 1 year of diagnosis,
- shortages of resources and staff within the registries,
- subjects unavailable for study because of involvement in other research studies, and
- adherence to physician and patient consent legal requirements being labor intensive (Baker, 1999).

The second survey is a cross-sectional study of 6,000 long-term survivors (i.e., those who are 2, 5, and 10 years beyond diagnosis) of 6 cancers (prostate, breast, colorectal, bladder, melanoma, uterine). The study design calls for 1,000 respondents for each type of cancer. The original study design included 15-year survivors, but relatively few registries were established in 1983 or earlier and had complete data necessary to identify 15-year survivors.

## DEVELOPING HEALTH SERVICES RESEARCH CONSORTIUMS

Many studies of cancer care quality exclude members of managed care organizations because such plans often do not have encounter data available (e.g., individual claims for visits or services). Such plans, however, cover the majority of privately insured Americans and have internal data systems available on the care of their members. A new initiative of the NCI, the Cancer Research Network (CRN), will encourage the expansion of collaborative cancer research among healthcare provider organizations that are oriented to community care; have access to large, stable, and diverse patient populations; and are able to take advantage of existing integrated databases that can provide patient-level information relevant to research studies on cancer control and to cancer-related population studies. Beginning in 1999, NCI funded the first CRN—a consortium of 10 large, not-for-profit, research-oriented HMOs. The CRN will conduct four main projects (Brown, 1999):

---

[2]The cancer sites include: prostate, female breast, lung, colorectal, urinary bladder, non-Hodgkin's lymphoma, skin melanoma, uterine, kidney, and ovarian.

1. a study of tobacco control policies and programs and their relationship to patient smoking cessation rates, and an analysis of healthcare smoking-related costs;

2. a study of late-stage breast and invasive cervical cancer cases to elucidate the patient, provider, and system factors that contribute to preventing advanced disease;

3. a study of the effectiveness of the commonly used strategies of frequent mammography or prophylactic mastectomy, to prevent fatal breast cancer among women at increased risk for breast cancer; and

4. a test of methods for increasing the participation of HMO patients in cancer clinical trials.

The CRN infrastructure will include a data-coordinating center and expert teams to provide scientific input in the areas of biostatistics, health economics, survey measures, pharmaco-epidemiology, genetics, clinical trials management, and survivorship issues.

## FEDERAL HEALTH SURVEYS AND DATA

The federal government spends a considerable amount on statistical activities related to health—nearly a billion dollars alone on direct funding of major statistical programs within the Department of Health and Human Services (OMB, 2000). The results from surveys and other data collection activities provide national estimates of such health indicators as the prevalence of health conditions, the use of healthcare services, and healthcare expenditures. Federal agencies also support methodological research that has fostered the development of standardized survey instruments (e.g., patient satisfaction with health care) and techniques to improve data processing and analysis. Examples of federal health surveys include the National Health Interview Survey, the National Ambulatory Medical Care Survey (NAMCS), the National Hospital Discharge Survey, and the Medical Expenditure Panel Survey. Some surveys are conducted for certain populations (e.g., the Medicare Current Beneficiary Survey) while others are targeted to specific health conditions (e.g., the AIDS Cost and Services Utilization Study). National surveys have been invaluable in estimating the prevalence of cancer risk behaviors (e.g., smoking) and use of preventive health services (e.g., mammography use) but have not been as useful in treatment-related quality-of-care studies.

Federal surveys conducted of individuals are often very large, including members of as many as 50,000 households. Even so, the incidence of cancer is estimated to be under 1%, making it difficult to identify large numbers of recently diagnosed cases of any particular type of cancer. Household surveys exclude residents of institutions and therefore miss individuals with cancer who are in nursing homes, hospices, or other facilities. There are also limitations in self-reports of cancer. Evidence suggests, for example, that many individuals do not accurately report the occurrence of cancer or the type of cancer diagnosed (Bergmann et al., 1998; Chambers et al., 1976). When national surveys of healthcare providers or facilities (e.g., NAMCS) are conducted, similar problems occur, such as accruing a sufficient sample of individuals with cancer, obtaining sufficient information on stage of illness and comorbidity, and determining the indication for a procedure (e.g., curative vs. palliative surgery).

Investigators at ACS have analyzed the National Hospital Discharge Survey from 1988 to 1995 to describe patterns of use of inpatient surgical procedures for treating cancers of the lung, colon/rectum, prostate, and female breast, by age, gender, race, and geographic region (Wingo, 1999). The results are useful in assessing general trends in service use and in generating hypotheses on apparent disparities in use, but they are difficult to interpret because of the lack of information on cancer stage and indication for the procedures. In general, national health surveys are extremely useful in gauging progress toward goals established in the area of cancer control and prevention but have limited applications in assessing other aspects of the quality of cancer care.

Some surveys include a sufficient sample of cancer patients to make robust analyses possible. Health services researchers interested in end-of-life care issues, for example, have used two surveys sponsored by the National Center for Health Statistics (NCHS), the National Home and Hospice Care Survey and the National Mortality Followback Survey (NMFS) (www.cdc.gov/nchs). As part of the NMFS, nearly 23,000 1993 death certificates were sampled and next of kin interviewed on where the decedent's death occurred, use of health care during the last year of life, unmet health needs, and the quality of the last year of life (e.g., functional limitations, use of pain medication).

A valuable data resource with which to assess the quality of hospital care is the Healthcare Cost and Utilization Project (HCUP) of the Agency for Healthcare Research and Quality (AHRQ). HCUP includes two databases for health services research:

- the Nationwide Inpatient Sample includes inpatient data from a national sample of about 1,000 hospitals, and
- the State Inpatient Database covers inpatient care in community hospitals in 22 states that represent more than half of all U.S. hospital discharges.

The uniform data in HCUP make possible comparative studies of the use and cost of hospital care, including the effects of market forces on hospitals and the care they provide, variations in medical practice, and the use of services by special populations (www.ahrq.gov/data/hcup). Examples of cancer-related health services research using HCUP include an analysis of hospital characteristics associated with breast-conserving surgery (Johantgen et al., 1995) and a study of geographic variations in sphincter-sparing surgery rates in the treatment of rectal cancer (Morris, 1999). Analyses of the association between volume of services and short-term outcomes for specific procedures are also possible because the HCUP databases include all discharges for a given hospital, not just a sample of discharges.

## SUMMARY

One of the most productive strategies health services researchers have used to assess the quality of cancer care has been to link cancer registry data to either administrative claims records or hospital discharge files. The data sources are often complementary—cancer registry data contain important information on diagnosis and cancer stage but may not record complete information on treatment that occurs outside the hospital. Administrative data may lack the diagnostic information but record a patient's treatment encounters. Linked data sets are not without problems. Administrative records may have treatments miscoded, comorbidity data needed to adjust results may be limited, and data elements necessary for complete linkage may be absent. Nevertheless, such linkages have allowed researchers to study variation in cancer care and to make comparisons across systems of care. A large study being conducted in California will provide information on the quality of registry treatment data, as well as maximize the potential of linkage using the cancer registry, hospital discharge data, and claims data from the Medicare program.

Many cancer registries are achieving nearly complete levels of case ascertainment, making them valuable as sampling frames for targeted special studies. Here, cancer registry staff may be asked to gather from medical charts clinical information to supplement that obtained for routine registry purposes. With appropriate resources, special studies can be launched relatively quickly in response to a specific research question. The SEER program has conducted a number of special studies, including a recent study of quality-of-life issues among men with prostate cancer following prostatectomy. The American Cancer Society is piloting two cancer survivorship surveys using state registries as sampling frames. Some state laws regarding confidentiality and consent have made timely access to research subjects difficult (e.g., requiring consent from the patient and the attending physician). Furthermore, Institutional Review Boards within hospitals can take several months to approve research projects.

The majority of privately insured Americans receive care within managed care organizations, but data on their care are often difficult to obtain because individual claims are usually not filed for each encounter. A number of plans have internal information systems and a population-based orientation to health care, making them ideal partners for research. The NCI has developed a consortium of such large managed care plans to collaborate on research.

Many of the federally sponsored national surveys can provide important descriptive information relevant to cancer, for example, use of health services and trends in service use. However, such surveys generally have limitations for cancer-related health services research because of the relatively rare occurrence of incident cases of disease and the lack of clinical detail on cancer (e.g., stage). Certain national data collection efforts, however, have great potential for cancer-related health services research. AHRQ's HCUP, for example, can be used to assess variations in patterns of care and differences in care across systems of care.

# 5

# Status of the Cancer Care Data System

The National Cancer Policy Board (board) has defined several characteristics of an ideal cancer care data system. The system should include meaningful indicators of care quality and provide quality benchmarks for use by systems of care (e.g., hospitals, provider groups, and managed care systems). The system should include recently diagnosed individuals with cancer in care settings representative of contemporary practice across the country, as well as draw from information sources with sufficient detail to allow appropriate comparisons. Chapter 2 described 10 attributes of an ideal system (which could include several distinct databases):

1. a set of well-established quality-of-care measures,
2. reliance on computer-based patient records for information on patient care and outcomes,
3. standard reporting of cancer stage, comorbidity, and processes of care,
4. national, population-based case selection,
5. repeated cross sectional studies to monitor national trends,
6. established benchmarks for quality improvement,
7. data systems for local quality assurance purposes,
8. public reporting of selected aggregate quality scores,
9. adaptability, and
10. protections to ensure privacy of health information.

This chapter evaluates how close we are to having such an ideal cancer care data system and discusses how progress could be made to achieve these attributes.

## WELL-ESTABLISHED QUALITY-OF-CARE MEASURES

In its April 1999 report, the board noted the absence of a core set of quality measures for cancer care and recommended that such a set be developed through a coordinated public–private effort. While there is no accepted set of measures, several "process" quality measures have been used to assess cancer care (Table 5.1). Process quality refers to what providers do for patients and how well they do it, both technically and interpersonally. Effective process measures are identified through evidence from appropriately designed studies (e.g., clinical trials) that show a link between a particular process of care and better outcomes. Once this link has been established, systems can be put into place to monitor adher-

**TABLE 5.1** Examples of Process Measures Used to Assess Quality of Cancer Care

| Cancer Site | Process Measure |
|---|---|
| Breast | Quality of staging information (tumor size, estrogen receptors, lymph node dissection) |
| | Initial biopsy prior to total mastectomy |
| | Use of breast conserving surgery for local disease |
| | Local breast radiation following lumpectomy |
| | Adjuvant chemotherapy for premenopausal women with node-positive cancer |
| | Use of perioperative bone scan (not indicated) |
| | Use of perioperative abdominal CT scan (not indicated) |
| | Referral to medical oncologist to discuss adjuvant therapy |
| | If mastectomy, visit to plastic surgeon to discuss reconstructive surgery |
| | Follow-up mammography within first 18 months post-operatively |
| | Follow-up bone or CT scans for suspicious symptoms per year (not indicated) |
| Colon | Adjuvant chemotherapy for Stage III disease |
| Rectum | Adjuvant chemotherapy and radiation therapy for Stage II/III disease |
| Prostate | Presentation of treatment alternatives to patient |
| | Rates of surgical treatment among men aged 70 and older (should be low) |
| Small-cell lung cancer (SCLC) | Chemotherapy for limited SCLC |
| Nonseminoma testicular cancer | Chemotherapy |
| Hodgkin's disease | Chemotherapy for Stage IIB or IV disease |
| Non-Hodgkin's lymphoma | Chemotherapy for diffuse intermediate or high-grade disease |

SOURCE: IOM, 1999a.

ence to the recommended processes. Current performance can be compared to a physician's or plan's prior performance, to the performance of other physicians and plans, or to benchmarks of performance. If performance falls below expected levels, educational or other interventions can be employed to change provider behavior.

Although they are intuitively appealing, measures of patient outcomes have certain limitations in the context of quality assessment. Many factors other than health care can affect outcomes; consequently, a finding of a higher-than-expected 5-year mortality rate in one hospital relative to another could just as easily reflect differences in patients' comorbidity status as the actual quality of care received. Process measures are advantageous because they tend to be frequent, immediate, controllable, and rarely confounded by other factors (Eddy, 1997). Some process measures, however, may depend on compliance or patient preferences. For example, although chemotherapy is highly recommended after surgery for certain cancers, some patients might decline treatment because they do not wish to experience its associated toxicities. Therefore, 100% adherence may not be a reasonable target for an indicator specifying adjuvant chemotherapy for these patients.

A set of "process" and "outcome" quality-of-care measures has been proposed for each phase of care for women with breast cancer (Mandelblatt et al., 1999) (Table 5.2). The authors of these proposed measures suggest that the measurement set be reviewed for its clinical relevance and feasibility, assessed for its validity and reliability, evaluated against established methodologic standards, and be subject to peer review.

Since the publication of the board's *Ensuring Quality Cancer Care* report, the National Cancer Institute (NCI) has committed to developing a core set of outcome measures. For each major cancer site, NCI plans to adopt, adapt, or develop one or more outcome measures applicable to each stage of the cancer care continuum, from prevention through end-of-life care (NCI, 1999b). NCI has commissioned several literature reviews to support this effort. NCI will also collaborate with the Agency for Healthcare Research and Quality (AHRQ, formerly the Agency for Health Care Policy and Research) to support and fund research aimed at increasing the use of guideline information in practice, for example, developing Web-based decision support tools for guideline development. NCI-sponsored research will also support evaluations of how such tools increase the likelihood that appropriate care is delivered to patients (NCI, 1999b).

Other efforts under way to define cancer care measures include the National Committee for Quality Assurance's (NCQA) appointment of an Oncology Measurement Advisory Panel to review measures relevant to cancer care (Oncology News, 1999; Winn, 1999). NCQA accredits managed care plans and has produced a widely used report card monitoring system called the Health Plan Employer Data and Information Set (HEDIS®) (www.ncqa.org). The HEDIS® cancer quality indicators have thus far targeted early detection and diagnosis, not care received after cancer is diagnosed. NCQA has implemented treatment-related quality measures for other conditions (e.g., diabetes) and has experience evaluating the feasibility of instituting a measure taking into consideration statistical issues involving sampling, the reliability of available clinical sources of information, and ensuring that valid comparisons can be made between health plans.

The American Society of Clinical Oncology (ASCO) is also planning to define a set of measures of quality of care to use in the development of a quality monitoring system for cancer patients (ASCO, 2000).

Health services research is also advancing in this area. Cancer quality indicators have, for example, recently been identified for six cancer sites (breast, cervical, colorectal, lung, prostate, skin) as part of a comprehensive quality measurement system designed to assess quality within managed care plans (Malin et al., 2000).

While first steps to identify and adopt cancer care measures are being taken within the cancer care community, a broadly focused response to issues of healthcare quality is taking shape at the federal level. In the wake of the influential report of the President's Advisory Commission on Consumer Protection and Quality in the Health Care Industry (1998), complementary bodies have been formed on healthcare quality—one in the public sector to promote interagency coordination among the Department of Health and Human Services (DHHS) and other federal agencies (Quality Interagency Coordination Task Force [QuIC]), and the other in the private sector to improve healthcare quality, measurement, and reporting (National Forum for Health Care Quality Measurement and Reporting [forum]). The aims and activities of both the QuIC and the forum are quite relevant to the quality cancer care agenda.

The QuIC's goal is to ensure that all federal agencies involved in purchasing, providing, studying, or regulating healthcare services are working in a coordinated way toward the common goal of improving quality of care. The Secretary of Health and Human Services and the Secretary of Labor serve as the co-chairs of the QuIC, and the Administrator of the Agency for Healthcare Research and Quality serves as the chairman for day-to-day operations. The QuIC seeks to (www.ahrq.gov/qual/quicfact.htm):

- provide people with information to assist them in making choices about their care,
- improve the care delivered by federal providers and purchased on behalf of federal beneficiaries, and
- develop the infrastructure need to improve the healthcare system.

The QuIC has established work groups in five areas:

1. *Patient and consumer information*—to address critical barriers to effective communication with patients about quality;

2. *Improving quality measurement*—to develop a "tool box" of quality measures and risk adjustment methods used by federal agencies (the work group is developing an inventory of measures and risk adjustment methods for use within federal agencies);

**TABLE 5.2** Potential Measures of the Quality of Breast Cancer Care

| Care Domain | Potential Measure | Process | Outcome | Data Source |
|---|---|---|---|---|
| Screening | Mammography rate (initial and return) | ✓ | | Administrative database, chart |
| | Clinical examination rates | ✓ | | Chart, patient self-report |
| | Stages of cancer | | ✓ | Chart, tumor registry |
| Diagnosis | Time from abnormal screen to diagnosis | ✓ | | Chart, administrative data |
| | Estrogen/progesterone receptors | ✓ | | Chart, laboratory, pathology reports |
| | Rate of true-positive biopsies | | ✓ | Chart, administrative data |
| Treatment, local and systemic | Documentation of choice for local and systemic treatment; documentation of patient participation | ✓ | | Chart, patient self-report |
| | Pain and symptom control | ✓ | | Chart, patient self-report |
| | Time from diagnosis to treatment | ✓ | | Administrative data |
| | Rate of tamoxifen prescription or chemotherapy | ✓ | | Chart, pharmacy data |
| | Offer of reconstruction/plastic surgery referral after mastectomy | ✓ | | Chart |

| | | | | |
|---|---|---|---|---|
| | Functional status/Quality of life | | ✓ | Patient survey, chart |
| | Satisfaction | | ✓ | Patient report |
| | Disease-free survival, survival | | ✓ | Chart |
| Rehabilitation | Evaluation of psychosocial needs | ✓ | | Chart, administrative data |
| | Rehabilitation evaluation | ✓ | | Chart, administrative data |
| | Psychologic function | | ✓ | Patient survey, chart |
| | Physical function | | ✓ | Patient survey, chart |
| Surveillance | Documentation of recurrence; rates of mammography and clinical breast exam | ✓ | | Chart |
| Palliative care | Pain control; offer of hospice; documentation of discussion of "Do Not Resuscitate" orders and living wills | ✓ | | Chart, patient report |
| | Quality of dying experience | | ✓ | Patient/family report |

SOURCE: Mandelblatt et al., 1999.

3. *Developing the workforce*—to determine how to expand and improve the current methods of ensuring the skills of the healthcare workforce, and equipping healthcare workers to improve the care they deliver;

4. *Key opportunities for improving clinical quality*—to mount an effort to improve clinical quality of care in two areas, diabetes and depression. For diabetes, the work group is focusing its efforts on having all federal programs agree to use the Diabetes Quality Indicator Project measures of care and then to improve healthcare provider performance based on these indicators. For depression, the work group is developing an evidence-based guideline to improve the identification and treatment of depressed individuals served by federal healthcare programs;

5. *Improving information systems*—to further efforts to develop a standardized language that will enable computerized comparisons of quality across federal agencies, and to examine the potential uses of telemedicine for helping to improve the quality of care.

The complementary Quality Forum established with a private-sector base will attempt to (http://www.qualityforum.org):

- ensure system-wide capacity to evaluate and report on the quality of care,
- promote and inform consumer choice and further consumer understanding and use of quality measures,
- enable providers to use data to improve performance,
- allow meaningful quality comparisons of healthcare providers and plans,
- promote competition on the quality of healthcare services,
- use broad representation to marshal market forces for quality, and
- reduce the burdens on providers and health plans by enabling them to collect consistent data that avoids duplication.

The board is encouraged that first steps toward the development of a core set of cancer care quality measures have been taken, and it hopes that its vision of a public/private collaboration on its creation will be realized. The mechanisms for such a collaboration appear to be in place.

## COMPUTER-BASED PATIENT RECORDS

The revolution in information technology provides many opportunities to improve the quality and timeliness of quality-of-care studies. Recording patient data using computer-based patient records (CPRs), Internet (and Intranet) communications, and statistical software provides opportunities to rapidly turn raw data into meaningful reports. The healthcare industry, however, lags behind others in adopting information technology that could promote faster feedback to providers on the quality of care (IOM workshop on Healthcare Informatics,

1999). For example, while all financial transactions are now electronic, relatively few health systems have CPR systems (www.himss.org/survey). A very sophisticated oncology patient record system has been developed for physicians practicing within the OnCare system (see Chapter 3). Here, physicians enter information into the CPR as they provide care. Embedded in the system are clinical practice guidelines, information on standard chemotherapy regimens, and summary data on the experience of other patients throughout the system available in near real time. Such systems are not yet in common use, and while promising, their impact on quality of care has not been fully evaluated.

While consumers are navigating the Internet in record numbers searching for information about their health and care, only 37% of office-based physicians were estimated to be using the World Wide Web in 1999 (www.ama-assn. org/ad-com/releases/1999/991203b.htm). This trend may change as new Internet-based products designed to ease the burden of filing insurance claims are targeted to physicians, and as medical professionals become more aware of informational resources provided via Internet access. Until physicians increase their use, the potential for the Internet or Intranets (controlled-access versions of the Internet) to improve the timeliness of reporting between clinicians and cancer registries will not be met. A major barrier to the adoption of information technology in medicine is concern about protecting the privacy of confidential medical information (see discussion below).

## STANDARD REPORTING

Quality assessments depend on the accurate recording of cancer stage and degree of comorbidity because what is considered appropriate treatment varies by these patient attributes. These factors must be carefully controlled when comparing the quality of care (e.g., by site of care, type of provider) so that apparent differences in quality can be correctly attributed to differences in attributes of care, rather than to differences in the degree of illness of the patients being compared.

### Cancer Stage

Three major staging systems are used for cancer surveillance in the United States: summary stage (SS); extent of disease (EOD); and tumor, node, metastasis (TNM). In addition, a number of site-specific staging schemes (e.g., prostate and bladder cancer, melanoma) are available. Within a particular staging system, different assignments also can be made, depending on whether one considers information from the pathology report or information from the patient's clinical assessment. This variation further complicates the staging options.

Cancer cases are often reported to multiple organizations, each with a preferred staging system. These varying expectations are burdensome for the person reporting the case. Furthermore, analysts who try to integrate these multiple sources of information, or who want to make comparisons across data systems, may have difficulty collapsing staging categories in one system to match another. Even within states, hospitals vary on how they report stage. Summary stage is used by most population-based registries, but clinical researchers do not find this measure to be sufficiently precise to evaluate the quality of care.

To address these issues, a Stage Task Force was established in 1997 to recommend a "best" staging system (Edge et al., 1999).[1] However, organizations resisted switching to a single staging system because of their various orientations and needs (e.g., historical trend analyses, evaluations of appropriateness of care). Consequently, the Task Force has instead recommended a uniform set of data items from which SS, EOD, and TNM can be derived. This uniform data collection set would likely ease the burden of reporting because one system with a single set of rules would be applicable for all organizations. Organizations that wanted to report data using their preferred system could use a computer algorithm to translate from the new uniform system back to any one of the other systems (i.e., SS, EOD, TNM).

## Comorbidity

The majority of cancer patients are over age 65 and often have ailments other than cancer. These conditions may render an overall prognosis so poor for the patient that an otherwise recommended treatment might be withheld. Furthermore, some comorbid conditions may affect patients' ability to tolerate recommended treatment for cancer, negatively affecting their response to treatment. Incorrect conclusions could be reached about the quality of care without sufficient information about comorbidity (Greenfield et al., 1988). Lower than expected use of a recommended cancer treatment at a particular hospital, for example, could signal a patient population too ill to tolerate the treatment, rather than the receipt of poor quality care.

Several instruments have been developed to classify different comorbid diseases and to quantify the severity of the overall comorbid condition (e.g., Charlson Comorbidity Index, Kaplan-Feinstein Index). None of the instruments were specifically designed to study comorbidity in cancer patients. Nevertheless, these instruments have been used to classify comorbidity in several types of cancers and have performed well (Piccirillo, 1999).

Very accurate assessments of comorbidity can be made with information from medical records, and recommendations have been made to train cancer registrars to code comorbidity and to include this information as a required data element in cancer registries (Piccirillo, 1999). In a pilot study, trained registrars could accurately and quickly code cases using a comorbidity index while they

---

[1]The Task Force is a collaboration of the American Joint Committee on Cancer (AJCC), the National Cancer Institute, the Centers for Disease Control and Prevention, and the North American Association of Central Cancer Registries (Edge et al., 1999).

abstracted information from the medical chart (Piccirillo et al., 1999). Somewhat less accurate and complete assessments of comorbidity can be made using claims data (e.g., Medicare hospital discharge summaries).

In addition to having standardized reporting of important clinical determinants of treatments and outcomes, information has to be available within a relatively short period of time, allowing for timely assessments of care. In its review of the literature on the quality of cancer care in *Ensuring Quality Cancer Care*, the board noted that many recently published studies relied upon the experience of patients cared for in the 1980s. In part, this observation reflects the inclusion in some research of a 5-year mortality outcome that, by definition, slows the reporting of results. One of the advantages of quality assessments that rely on process of care measures is the more rapid turnaround time for results.

## NATIONAL, POPULATION-BASED CASE SELECTION

Almost all of the case studies of quality care assessment described in Chapter 3 relied on convenience samples of patients. The initiative at Roswell Park Cancer Institute, for example, identified cancer cases through one insurance company's claims. This quality assessment was cosponsored by the insurer, and the intention of the study was to assess the quality of care delivered to that defined population. The convenience sampling employed was therefore entirely consistent and appropriate given the aims of the study. Indeed, quality studies are probably most appropriately conducted through health systems responsible for the care of the group of patients under study. Within these circumstances, results are more likely to be acted upon by administrators and providers.

Broad-based assessments, however, are needed to determine the quality of care nationally and to understand if certain population subgroups are particularly subject to substandard care. Furthermore, the establishment of national benchmarks of care that can be used by local systems of care to evaluate their programs relative to others in their area, or to the population as a whole, depend on samples that are nationally, or at least regionally, representative. Notable in almost all of the case studies was the lack of comparison values on measures applied within the studies. Currently, no national benchmarks of the quality of cancer care exist.

The source with the greatest promise for delivering representative samples of patients with which to measure the quality of cancer care is the state cancer registries, recently organized into the National Program of Cancer Registries (NPCR). Other potential sources include the Surveillance, Epidemiology, and End Results (SEER) program of the NCI, and the National Cancer Data Base (NCDB), cosponsored by the American College of Surgeons' Commission on Cancer (ACoS-CoC) and the American Cancer Society (ACS) (also described in Chapter 3).

## National Program of Cancer Registries

In all states, cancer is a reportable disease; that is, by law it must be reported to a state registry (J. Enders, acting section chief, Cancer Surveillance Branch, CDC, personal communication, March 30, 2000; www.cdc.gov/nccdphp).[2] Registries are essential to understanding the burden of cancer and in evaluating the success of cancer prevention programs. They are also used to target resources to areas that may be underserved by screening or public health education programs. The central purpose of state cancer registries is cancer surveillance, monitoring the burden of cancer for a given population.

When registration activities are organized to obtain complete counts of cancer for a given population (e.g., a state), the system is said to be "population-based" (Austin, 1994). Some registries focus on developing incident rates, the rate of new cases of cancer for their population. Such "incidence only" registries must have accurate and complete case counts and the data necessary to categorize patients and tumors. The need for, and the success of, cancer control programs can be assessed with these registries. Other population-based registries have a broader charge and may follow up on cases identified to collect data on outcomes (e.g., recurrence, death) and treatment. These registries are able to provide information on survival rates among those diagnosed with cancer and to address issues regarding access to certain cancer care services.

Cancer registries strive to identify at least 90% of new cases of cancer within 2 years after the diagnosis year and maintain a high degree of accuracy as determined by the North American Association of Centralized Cancer Registries (NAACCR) certification process (Tucker et al., 1999). In 1999, NAACCR certified 19 U.S. population-based state registries as having achieved this level of quality (Appendix D). The draft *Healthy People 2010* objectives for cancer surveillance include "Increas[ing] the number of states that have a statewide population-based cancer registry that captures case information on at least 95% of the expected number of reportable cancers" (M. Kaiser, Office of Program and Policy Information, NCCDPHP, CDC, personal communication, January 19, 2000).

The cancer registration process is very labor intensive, and registries may not report on cases ascertained in a given year for 2 to 3 years. It can take this long to complete data collection on identified cases, for example, those residing in one state but diagnosed and treated in another. Extensive time may also be needed to obtain information on those reported to the registry by private pathology laboratories. Private laboratories may not provide necessary identifying information on the patient for whom the diagnosis was made (i.e., the registry may have to contact the physician who referred the specimen for analysis).

---

[2]While all states have some form of mandated cancer reporting, the degree to which reporting is required varies. Most states require reporting from all acute care hospitals, but others require more extensive reporting (e.g., from outpatient surgery/treatment centers, pathology labs, or physician offices) (J. Enders, acting section chief, Cancer Surveillance Branch, CDC, personal communication, March 30, 2000).

Identifying duplicate records and consolidating their respective information can also delay the process. A cancer patient could be reported to the registry multiple times, for example, first by the surgeon, then by the oncologist. A single case record needs to be constructed to reflect the experience of the patient as recorded in each report. While the cancer registration process is a lengthy one, rapid case ascertainment is possible for special studies so that investigators can quickly gather information on identified study subjects (e.g., within a month of diagnosis) (Aldrich et al., 1995).

Responding to the needs of states, Congress established the NPCR in 1992 (Cancer Registries Amendment Act, P.L. 102-515) and authorized the Centers for Disease Control and Prevention (CDC) to administer the program. At that time, 10 states had no central cancer registry. The remaining states had registries operating at some level, but many lacked the financial support and personnel to gather complete, timely, and accurate data on their population and to ensure that the data collected met CDC's minimum standards of quality (DHHS, CDC, *1999 NPCR at-a-Glance*). Since 1994, the CDC has bolstered state efforts to improve cancer registration through the NPCR. With fiscal year 1999 appropriations of approximately $24 million, the CDC supported 45 states, 3 territories, and the District of Columbia for cancer registries.[3] Costs are shared with registries, with the CDC covering 75% and the state covering 25% of the costs (total expenditure is $32 million). In addition to financial assistance, the CDC provides technical assistance to states (e.g., computerized reporting and data processing systems, model legislation for statewide cancer registries) and has established program standards and a monitoring system to assess data completeness, timeliness, and quality (Chen et al., 1999; DHHS, 1999; Penman et al., 1996). Once states meet NPCR standards, plans are for state data to be combined into a database that will be made available to public health practitioners and cancer researchers. With additional appropriations, CDC would help states link their cancer registries with other data sets to:

- improve the quality of the registry (e.g., through linkages with the National Death Index),
- facilitate epidemiological research (e.g., through linkages with census data and geographic information systems), and
- permit health services research (e.g., through linkage with administrative records of the Health Care Financing Administration [HCFA]).

Once the state registries reach established NPCR standards, NPCR (together with SEER) has great potential to support efforts to monitor the quality of cancer care. When data from state registries are pooled, virtually all of the nation's cancer cases will be included in one database. The registries by themselves are

---

[3]The five state registries funded through SEER do not receive support from the NPCR.

not sufficient for comprehensive assessments of quality of care. Information on the first course of treatment is generally collected by state registries, but treatments provided outside the reporting facility are underreported (Bickell and Chassin, 2000). There are, however, great opportunities for learning about the quality of cancer care through linkages to other sources, such as hospital discharge files or claims for hospital and outpatient care from the Medicare program or private insurers. Examples of health services research using state registry data published in the last 10 years are summarized in Appendix C. A study being conduced in California will help evaluate the strengths and limitations of using a state cancer registry to answer questions about the quality of cancer care (described in Chapter 4) (Ayanian, 1999).

State cancer registry data are limited as far as studies of cancer care quality are concerned. The registries were not originally intended to serve this function, but data elements have been added in some states to facilitate quality studies. Identified limitations of cancer registry data for quality studies include (Weeks, 1999):

- limited treatment data (e.g., chemotherapy drugs/regimens not specified),
- information on treatment delivered in physician's offices largely missing,
- no information on comorbidity,
- no data on use of diagnostic procedures,
- outcomes data limited to recurrence and survival,
- lag time in data availability up to 2 years, and
- limited resources within registries for analyses.

On the other hand, state registry data have some strengths (Ayanian, 1999):

- inclusive population-based cohorts,
- information about the tumor (e.g., stage, site, histology, grade),
- nearly complete demographic data, and
- data can be linked to Census, Medicare, and hospital discharge data.

The ACS, in collaboration with the American College of Surgeons and three state cancer registries (Illinois, Kentucky, Louisiana), is evaluating the completeness and quality of treatment data for patients with colon cancer. Different approaches to collecting data from both hospital and outpatient settings will be assessed with the aim of estimating the proportion of colon cancer patients who receive optimal treatment, given the stage of their disease at diagnosis. Data acquired in a more timely fashion could be used by clinicians, individual hospitals, and state health department officials as benchmarks to gauge the quality of care provided. Success in this feasibility study could lead to the study of other cancer sites in additional states (P. Wingo, Department of Epidemiology and Surveillance Research, American Cancer Society, personal communication, October 1999).

## The Surveillance, Epidemiology, and End Results
## (SEER) Program

The SEER program is a system of population-based registries administered since 1973 by NCI (NCI/SIG, 1999). The NCI contracts with organizations in five states (Connecticut, Iowa, New Mexico, Utah, and Hawaii) and six metropolitan areas (Detroit, San Francisco/Oakland, Seattle/Puget Sound, San Jose/Monterey, Atlanta, Los Angeles) around the country to collect information on all new cases of cancer diagnosed in their geographic areas. Two supplemental registries were added to increase representation of American Indians and rural African Americans. Cases are followed up annually to determine survival. These data, along with data on cancer-related deaths from the National Center for Health Statistics (NCHS), are analyzed to provide incidence, mortality, and survival rate estimates for the entire country.

The SEER program represents the "gold" standard for cancer registration in the United States. The SEER registries have an extensive quality assurance program (e.g., case-finding audits, education and training of personnel), and the result is near complete ascertainment of cases (98%) and follow-up (95% of cases). The resources needed to achieve this level of success are estimated at approximately $150 per case (B. Hankey, chief, Cancer Statistics Branch, NCI, personal communication, September 22, 1999). The annual NCI budget for SEER is approximately $18 million. Costs are shared with registries, with NCI covering 80% and the registry covering 20% of the costs (total budget of about $22 million).

Information on the first course of treatment (e.g., surgery to primary site, radiation, chemotherapy) is recorded in SEER, but adjuvant therapies are not. In general, the SEER data suffer the same problems as NPCR state registry data in terms of their stand-alone capacity to be used to answer questions about the quality of care (e.g., lack of information on comorbidity). The SEER data have, however, been an invaluable source of information about the quality of cancer care, through NCI's patterns of care studies, special studies, and linkages to Medicare files (see Chapter 4).

The CDC and NCI have recently agreed to increase their level of collaboration in several areas, including: expansion of the SEER program (to include some NPCR registries); use of NPCR data to assess regional and national cancer rates; providing of data for public use; sponsorship of registry-related training activities; and conduct of research (DHHS, PHS, 2-14-00).

## The National Cancer Data Base

ACoS-CoC, in collaboration with ACS, cosponsors NCDB, a repository of cancer reports from 1,500 hospitals and other facilities in all 50 states (Morrow, 1999). In 1997, 873,000 cases, representing roughly 69% of the nation's cancer cases, were reported to NCDB (Stewart, personal communication, May 15, 2000). Estimates now suggest that NCDB includes as many as 80% of cases (M. Morrow, professor of surgery, Northwestern Medical Hospital, personal communication, January 5 and April 10, 2000) (the NCDB is also described in Chapter 3, as Case Study 10). Missing from NCDB are cases diagnosed and managed in community-based private practice office settings (e.g., many cases of melanoma, prostate cancer). For many cancers, ascertainment is nearly complete because diagnosis and initial treatment are almost always hospital based (e.g., colorectal cancer). The Commission on Cancer has reporting requirements that are somewhat different than those for the NPCR-funded registries or for SEER. NCDB, for example, collects information on diagnosis (e.g., TNM staging) and treatment (e.g., surgical approach, reconstructive/restorative procedures) not required of NPCR or SEER (Appendix E).

## Summary

The three national sources of data on cancer just described have some common elements. They all, for example, contain hospital-reported cases of cancer, but they are different in most other respects (Table 5.3). Whereas NPCR and SEER are focused on surveillance, NCDB was designed as a tool with which to monitor the quality of cancer care. NPCR and NCDB are national in scope, while the SEER registry is limited to a few geographic areas. When fully operational, NPCR (together with SEER) has the potential of being a truly national cancer surveillance system. Many fewer cases are processed each year by SEER, and resources are focused on ensuring that the quality of data is high. NPCR and SEER are population-based, and rates of cancer can be derived for their respective coverage areas. In contrast, NCDB is largely limited to hospital-reported cases, and certain patients and types of cancer are known to be under-represented (e.g., patients diagnosed and cared for in community-based private practice office settings, such as those with prostate cancer or melanoma) (Karagas et al., 1991; Koh et al., 1991). Because NCDB was designed to assess the quality of care, it contains more data elements collected on treatment than is the case for either NPCR or SEER.

While the purposes and coverage properties of the programs differ, significant overlap occurs across programs. In some areas, the same case of cancer appears in each data file. A registrar working in a hospital within a SEER area would need to complete three reports for a newly diagnosed patient with cancer, one for each of these programs. Each report would differ somewhat according to the reporting specifications of the respective programs. The reporting of stage of disease differs, as does the detail on demographic characteristics (e.g., ethnicity) and the details of cancer treatment (see Appendix E for a detailed description of reporting requirement of the three programs). It is very difficult to estimate the total cost of collecting cancer data. Federal and state contributions for the NPCR and SEER program total 54 million, but this excludes the high costs of reporting cases that are borne by hospitals, physicians, and other providers that report cancer cases.

**TABLE 5.3** Characteristics of Three Cancer Data Programs—NPCR, SEER, NCDB

| Characteristic | NPCR | SEER | NCDB |
|---|---|---|---|
| Purpose | Surveillance | Surveillance | Quality of care |
| Sponsor | Centers for Disease Control and Prevention | National Cancer Institute | American College of Surgeons' Commission on Cancer; American Cancer Society |
| Financial support* | $32 million per year (75% CDC; 25% State) | $22 million per year (80% NCI; 20% State) | $1.2 million per year |
| Geographic coverage | National, except 5 SEER states | Limited (5 states, 6 metro areas) | National |
| Population-based | Yes | Yes | No |
| Source of cases | Hospitals MD offices/clinics Pathology labs Out-of-state registries Death certificates | Hospitals MD offices/clinics Pathology labs Out-of-state registries Death certificates | Hospitals |
| Cases/records added annually | Roughly 1 million | 160,000 | 873,000 |
| Treatment data | First course only | First course only | First course, surgical detail, reconstructive procedures, biological response modifier therapy |
| Data availability | Through NAACCR | Public-use files | No |

*Costs associated with data collection are borne by the reporting facilities.

SOURCES: DHHS 2000; B. Hankey, chief, Cancer Statistics Branch, NCI, personal communication, September 22, 1999; Morrow, 1999; NCI/SIG, 1999.

With the diversity of programs and reporting standards, a number of organizations have been formed to facilitate communication, coordination, and standardization:

• *National Coordinating Council for Cancer Surveillance* (NCCCS) includes representation from ACS, ACoS-CoC, NCI, CDC, National Cancer Registrars Association, and NAACCR. The NCCCS was established to provide a forum for communication with an aim to improve the measurement of incidence, mortality, morbidity, and survival (cancer management is outside of their purview) (Swan et al., 1998).

• *The North American Association of Central Cancer Registries* (NAACCR) establishes and maintains standards for cancer registration. It provides training and education in cancer registry operations and certifies registries that achieve standards of high quality. It aggregates data annually from population-based registries throughout the United States and Canada. Finally, it promotes the use of cancer registry data in surveillance, cancer control, and population-based research. (www.naaccr.org).

• *The International Association of Cancer Registries* (IACR), closely associated with the International Agency for Research on Cancer (IARC), is a membership organization of international cancer registries "concerned with the collection and analysis of data on cancer incidence and with the end results of cancer treatment in defined population groups" (Wagner, 1991).

NPCR, SEER, and NCDB have different orientations and purposes. From the perspective of quality assessment, each of the programs has specific strengths and weaknesses (Table 5.4). In terms of timeliness, NCDB has a quicker processing time because the cases that slow down population-based registry programs are excluded from it (e.g., cases reported from private laboratories with little information available on the patient). Cases identified in a single hospital can be reported out fairly quickly because the data necessary to complete reporting are generally in the medical chart. Cases from state registries can take from 2 to 3 years to process because information might have to be obtained from registries in other states or from death certificates.

As for being representative, the state registries are advantageous because they are population based and, when taken together, are nationally representative. SEER registries are population-based but are located in just a few states and metropolitan areas (14% of the population is covered by SEER). NCDB, in contrast, has some inherent biases in that the program is not population based, and certain types of patients and cancers are known to be underrepresented. Furthermore, there is likely some bias in the type of hospitals that report cases to NCDB. On the other hand, NCDB has many cases available for analysis, and the information available on these cases is likely of relatively high quality because most cases are reported from ACoS-CoC approved hospitals where quality assurance programs and a review of sample cases are required. Perhaps the greatest opportunities to assess quality lie with linkages to other sources of data. Here, both NPCR and SEER registry data have been linked to provide valuable insights into quality of care issues.

## ESTABLISHED BENCHMARKS FOR QUALITY IMPROVEMENT

A benchmark is something that serves as a standard by which others can be measured. As applied in the business world, benchmarking is the identification of industry leaders so that their practices may be understood and emulated (Kiefe et al., 1998). Benchmarks are integral to healthcare quality improvement initiatives but with few exceptions have not been established for cancer care. Methods to quantify "Achievable Benchmarks of Care" (ABC$^{TM}$) have been developed that are based on the performance of a group of peers according to "process of care" quality indicators (Kiefe et al., 1998). Benchmarks using this method were first developed for patients with acute myocardial infarction (AMI) in the Cooperative Cardiovascular Project, an initiative undertaken as part of HCFA's Health Care Quality Improvement Program. Benchmarks were established by first transforming published clinical guidelines into computerized algorithms and then analyzing patterns of care. The following process measures were used to develop benchmarks for AMI:

- smoking cessation counseling;
- aspirin, angiotensin converting enzyme-inhibitor, and Beta-blocker prescriptions at discharge; and
- aspirin and low-dose heparin administration during hospitalization.

Information was abstracted from medical records by the Peer Review Organizations (PROs) in pilot states. In Alabama, for example, there were 106 hospitals that had a total of 1,253 AMI patients who should have been counseled to stop smoking. The 106 hospitals were ranked in order of their smoking cessation counseling rates, and then enough hospitals were selected, from the top-ranked down, to include at least 10% of patients eligible for smoking cessation counseling (i.e., 125 patients). This process resulted in the selection of 12 hospitals as the high performance hospitals, or benchmark contributors. Pooling the patients eligible for counseling from these 12 hospitals resulted in a benchmark performance level of 49%. The method identifies benchmarks that represent excellence but should be attainable by others. Refinements of the methodology have been made to ensure that providers with high performance levels, but small numbers of cases, do not unduly influence the level of the benchmark.

The ABC$^{TM}$ benchmarking methodology has been successfully implemented in several quality improvement projects, focusing on diabetes mellitus, breast and cervical cancer screening, and stroke (Weissman et al., 1999). It has also been

TABLE 5.4 Strengths and Weaknesses of National Cancer Data Programs from the Perspective of Quality Monitoring

| Data System/ Sponsor/Focus | Coverage | Strengths | Weaknesses |
|---|---|---|---|
| **NPCR** CDC Designed for surveillance, recommended data elements established by NPCR (states vary in the collection of cancer treatment information) | State registries vary in their ability to capture incident cancer cases. In 1999, 14 NPCR and 5 SEER states were certified by NAACCR for having high quality 1996 incidence data (e.g., they identified at least 90% of cases) (see Appendix D). | Near national coverage Most states ascertaining at least 90% of incident cancer cases National standards for data collection Linkage to administrative records for quality-related health services research | Data are not available for 2–3 years following case ascertainment. The quality of data on treatment has yet to be fully evaluated. |
| **SEER** NCI Designed for surveillance, includes information on first course of treatment | Registry includes residents in 5 states (CT, IA, NM, UT, HI), 6 metro areas (San Francisco/Oakland, Los Angeles County, San Jose/Monterey area | High-quality data Linkage to Medicare administrative data, providing a resource for quality-related health services research. | Limited geographic coverage, not selected to be representative of U.S. population. Literature suggests that SEER areas are more affluent and more urban than other areas and have different healthcare characteristics (e.g., more |

| | | cancer specialists) (Nattinger et al., 1997). Age-adjusted mortality rates by race and sex sometimes differ for SEER areas as compared to the U.S. suggesting that the SEER coverage population is not representative of the greater U.S. population (Frey et al., 1992). Data are not available for 2–3 years following case ascertainment. |
|---|---|---|
| Detroit, Atlanta, Seattle), and 3 supplemental registries representing 14% of the U.S. population. Within these areas case ascertainment is over 95%. | | |
| **National Cancer Data Base**<br>American College of Surgeons/American Cancer Society<br>Designed to monitor quality of cancer care<br><br>In 1997, an estimated 69% of incident cancer cases were reported by 1,629 of 2,000 hospitals with tumor registries (81% of hospitals with registries). | A high proportion of incident cancers included nationally<br>Recurrence and survival outcomes tracked<br>Data available for analysis relatively soon after collection | Individuals not diagnosed or treated in hospitals are not represented (e.g., cancer, such as melanoma, treated in outpatient settings).<br>Relatively high response rate among selected hospitals, but there is potential for bias. |

applied to the determination of a target for population-based mammography screening rates; this target has been proposed as a realistic, data-driven goal for adoption in Healthy People 2010 (Allison, 1999). Once agreement on "process" measures for cancer care has been reached, this model developed for AMI could be tested among cancer care providers.

## DATA SYSTEMS FOR LOCAL
## QUALITY ASSURANCE PURPOSES

Once benchmarks are established, hospitals, health plans, and provider groups should be able to assess their care relative to national or regional norms and identify ways that care could be improved. Individual providers who are working within large systems, for example, an integrated delivery system, or who are caring for employees of big companies or subscribers of large insurers, may be subject to quality improvement programs. Experience suggests that once credible performance data are presented to providers, better clinical behavior and improved care will follow (Lazar and Desch, 1998; Newcomer, 1997).

An accountability framework is developing within the private sector, which incorporates performance measurement of health plans and other healthcare organizations. Inclusion of cancer care measures into these systems could provide valuable information about cancer care to consumers, purchasers, and providers of care:[*]

• Health plans report quality of care data to the National Committee on Quality Assurance (NCQA), an accrediting body for managed care plans.
• Hospitals and healthcare organizations are surveyed and accredited according to standards established by the Joint Commission on the Accreditation of Healthcare Organizations (JCAHO) and, since 1997, have been required to participate in a quality performance system.

In 1998, NCQA, JCAHO, and the American Medical Association established the Performance Measurement Coordinating Council, a 15-member group that will work to coordinate performance measurement activities across the entire healthcare system (www.jcaho.org).

### National Committee for Quality Assurance

NCQA accredits managed care plans, Health Maintenance Organizations (HMOs), and Preferred Provider Organizations (PPOs) (www.ncqa.org). NCQA has also produced a widely used report card monitoring system called HEDIS®. HEDIS® measures were initially designed to provide information to large pur-

---

[*]Cancer care quality assurance programs are described in detail in Chapter 6 of *Ensuring Quality Cancer Care* (IOM, 1999a).

chasers about the quality of care offered to employees. More recently, the audience for results from HEDIS® has broadened, and HEDIS® indicators are often reported in consumer-oriented report cards.

HEDIS® is a performance measurement tool designed to assist purchasers and consumers in evaluating managed care plans and holding plans accountable for the quality of their services. Because HEDIS® has standard measures and uniform data reporting requirements, comparisons can be made across various health plans and their organizational structures (e.g., staff-model HMOs, point-of-service plans). The most recent iteration, HEDIS® 2000, assesses plans in eight domains (www.ncqa.org):

- effectiveness of care,
- accessibility and availability of care,
- satisfaction with the experience of care,
- stability of the health plan,
- use of services,
- cost of care,
- informed healthcare choices, and
- descriptive information about the plan.

HEDIS® 2000 measures relevant to cancer care are shown in Box 5.1.

---

**BOX 5.1 Selected Cancer-Specific (or cancer-relevant) HEDIS® 2000 Measures**

**Effectiveness of Care**
- Advising smokers to quit
- Cervical cancer screening
- Breast cancer screening

**Access to or Availability of Care**
- Adults' access to preventive ambulatory health services
- Availability of language interpretation services

**Satisfaction with the Experience of Care**
- Member satisfaction

**Health Plan Stability**
- Disenrollment
- Practitioner turnover

**Health Plan Descriptive Information**
- Provider board certification or residency completion
- Practitioner compensation
- Arrangements with public health, educational, and social service organizations

SOURCE: www.ncqa.org, Accessed February 17, 2000.

The HEDIS® cancer quality indicators have targeted early detection and diagnosis, not care received after cancer is diagnosed. Treatment-related indicators are being evaluated, for example, assessment of the effect of breast cancer therapy on a woman's ability to function and patients' satisfaction with breast cancer treatment. NCQA has halted further work on the indicator related to the stage at which breast cancer is detected because the incidence of breast cancer cases in most health plans is too low to make meaningful comparisons of stage at diagnosis across health plans (Schuster et al., 1998a). NCQA has appointed an Oncology Measurement Advisory Panel to review quality measures relevant to cancer care.

HEDIS® is a voluntary system, although managed care plans are finding it increasingly necessary to participate to compete for patients. More than 90% of HMOs report HEDIS® measures, and about 65% of Fortune 500 employers use NCQA accreditation and HEDIS® measures to evaluate the managed care plans with which they contract (O'Kane, 2000). NCQA produces Quality Compass, a CD-ROM-based system that makes it possible for consumers to obtain comparative HEDIS® ratings for HMOs in communities throughout the United States. A subset of Quality Compass measures appears on the World Wide Web. A health plan can refuse to disclose its HEDIS® profile to the public. In 1997, less than half of plans (45%) permitted public reporting of the data (Bodenheimer, 1999).

## Joint Commission on the Accreditation of Healthcare Organizations

The nonprofit JCAHO, the oldest and largest standard-setting and accrediting body in health care, has broadened its institutional coverage from solely hospitals to a wide array of delivery systems, including health plans, integrated delivery networks, PPOs, home care organizations, nursing homes and other long-term care facilities, behavioral healthcare organizations, ambulatory care providers, and clinical laboratories. JCAHO evaluates and accredits more than 19,000 healthcare organizations in the United States (www.jcaho.org). About 80% of U.S. hospitals participate, representing about 96% of all inpatient admissions.

For accreditation, JCAHO conducts an on-site quality assessment every 3 years. It covers such topics as patient rights, patient care, patient education, continuity of care, ongoing efforts to improve quality, safety plans, information management, and infection control. Although JCAHO (and other accrediting organizations) has traditionally focused on structural measures of quality—such as whether a hospital has appropriate capacity for the covered patient population—it now incorporates process and outcomes measures into its accreditation criteria. JCAHO relies on ACoS-CoC survey findings for cancer programs within JCAHO-accredited organizations (www.facs.org/about_college/acsdept/cancer_dept/cocjcaho.html).

JCAHO instituted the ORYX system in 1997, which requires organizations seeking JCAHO accreditation to select from among 60 performance measurement systems and two specific indicators on which they will report their care. Hospitals and long-term care facilities began reporting with these indicators during early 1999. With institutions choosing their own indicators, making comparisons across institutions will be challenging. It should allow for comparisons with prior years within the same institution, benchmarks, and goals. One of the accepted indicator systems is the MEDSTAT Group's Indicator Measurement System (IMSystem®), which has specifications for 42 quality-of-care indicators (including 5 for cancer care, Table 5.4). About 20–25 hospitals currently use the IMSystem® oncology measures (L. Homra, clinical consultant, MEDSTAT Group, personal communication, February 17, 2000).

## Public Reporting of Aggregate Quality Scores

The board has recommended that "Cancer care quality measures should be disseminated widely and communicated to purchasers, providers, consumer organizations, individuals with cancer, policy makers, and health services researchers, in a form that is relevant and useful for healthcare decision-making" (IOM, 1999a). Quality measures enable consumers and purchasers to judge the quality of a system of care by its performance relative to evidence-based standards. Many opportunities are available for exerting leverage on the healthcare system to improve quality:

• Large employer groups are holding managed care plans accountable for quality performance goals.
• HCFA requires Medicare and Medicaid health plans to produce standard quality reports.
• State Medicaid programs are beginning to include quality provisions in their contracts with plans and providers.

Six of 10 new cancer cases occur among people aged 65 and older and, consequently, Medicare is the principal payer for cancer care. The number of evaluations of the quality of care among Medicare beneficiaries will increase because breast cancer has been identified as one of six conditions that state-based PROs must now target in their efforts to improve the quality of care (Jencks, 1999).

Information about quality cancer care is becoming more available to individuals with cancer (or at risk for cancer), but it is not yet easily accessible or understandable by consumers. By the time a diagnosis of cancer is made and individuals have a clear reason to seek quality care, it is often too late to switch health plans. Also, even if they wanted to switch, most people do not have access to alternative plans. Individuals may use available quality indicators to choose doctors and hospitals within their plans, and perhaps to choose alternative courses of treatment, but evidence suggests that individual consumers can exert only a modest "market" pressure for quality improvement through access

**TABLE 5.4** IMSystem® Oncology Indicators

| | Data | Staging | Breast Cancer | Lung Cancer | Colon or Rectum Cancer |
|---|---|---|---|---|---|
| Focus | Availability of data for diagnosis and staging | Use of staging by managing physicians | Use of tests critical for prognosis and clinical management of female breast cancer | Effectiveness of preoperative diagnosis and staging | Comprehensiveness of diagnostic workup |
| Numerator | Patients undergoing resection for primary cancer of the lung, colon or rectum, or female breast for whom a surgical pathology consultation report is present in the medical record | Patients undergoing resection for primary cancer of the lung, colon or rectum, or female breast with stage of tumor designated by a managing physician | Female patients with Stage I or greater primary breast cancer who, after initial biopsy or resection, have estrogen receptor analysis results in the medical record | Patients with non-small-cell primary lung cancer undergoing thoracotomy with complete surgical resection of tumor | Patients undergoing resection for primary cancer of the colon or rectum whose preoperative evaluation by a managing physician included examination of the entire colon |
| Denominator | Patients undergoing resection for primary cancer of the lung, colon or rectum, or female breast | Patients undergoing resection for primary cancer of the lung, colon or rectum, or female breast | Female patients with Stage I or higher primary breast cancer undergoing initial biopsy or resection | Patients with non-small-cell primary lung cancer undergoing thoracotomy | Patients undergoing resection for primary cancer of the colon or rectum |

SOURCE: IMSystem,® 1997.

to better information about the quality of cancer care (IOM, 1999a). Large purchasers, such as employers, are likely to exert more leverage and to have designated staff to assess alternative plans.

A few purchasing coalitions are using information on cancer care quality to improve care (see Case Study 9 in Chapter 3). The Pacific Business Group on Health (PBGH), for example, is a nonprofit coalition of large healthcare purchasers in California and Arizona representing, as of 1996, 2.5 million insured individuals. PBGH collects and analyzes health plan performance data to produce report cards for consumers; promotes shared treatment decision making between providers and consumers; and collects, analyzes, and reports plan-level consumer satisfaction ratings (Castles et al., 1999; President's Advisory Commission, 1998). PBGH is also developing several disease-specific quality assessment programs, including one for breast cancer. PBGH was the first purchasing coalition to impose a condition on contracting plans whereby it would withhold 2% of the premium until the plans achieved specific goals for improving customer satisfaction and quality of care.

NCI is cofunding with AHRQ a Request for Proposals entitled "Making Quality Count." One of the areas of study that will be encouraged is the use of report cards and other tools for communicating quality of care information to payers, providers, and patients. Innovation and research in the presentation of this information will also be sought (NCI, 1999b). NCI also plans to conduct a national cancer communications survey, which will have a quality of cancer care module to assess how people obtain quality of care information, and what their preferences are for this type of information. NCI will also develop and issue an RFA for fiscal year 2001 to create cancer communications "centers of excellence." Prospective applicants will be encouraged to focus, in part, on quality-of-care issues.

## Protections to Ensure Privacy of
## Health Information

Legal protections and data security systems must be in place to ensure that data collected and stored about an individual's diagnosis and treatment of cancer are used only for legitimate public health purposes. No legal action regarding a breach of confidentiality from cancer registries has been reported, but concerns about privacy[1] and confidentiality[2] are increasing as data are being transmitted electronically and cancer registry data are being merged with other sources (Coleman et al., 1992; Newcombe, 1995). Personal identifiers, including name, birth date, and social security number are required data elements in the NPCR and NCDB because effective cancer registration involves the collection and

---

[1]Health information privacy is an individual's claim to control the circumstances in which personally identifiable information is collected, used, and transmitted (Hodge, 1999).

[2]Confidentiality is privacy interests arising out of a specific relationship with the person about whom information is gathered (Hodge, 1999).

linkage of data about individuals with cancer, often from several different sources. Such linkages, for example, are necessary to eliminate duplicate reports of a case from different healthcare providers, and to identify deaths that have occurred among cases reported to the registry so that survival statistics can be calculated (linkage to death certificate data). Furthermore, data sharing must occur between states to identify residents diagnosed out-of-state. Even though the NPCR and NCDB require that social security number and other identifying information be reported when they are available, these data elements are not forwarded to a central entity at either the CDC or NCDB. Having personal identifiers available centrally could facilitate national or regional assessments of the quality of cancer care, but such use of personal identifying information raises a host of legal and ethical issues.

The CDC has provided model legislation for states to assist them in complying with provisions of the Cancer Registries Amendment Act of 1992 (the Act that established the NPCR). According to this act, states must promulgate regulations providing "for the protection of the confidentiality of all cancer case data reported to the statewide cancer registry, including a prohibition on disclosure to any person of information reported to the statewide cancer registry that identifies, or could lead to the identification of an individual cancer patient, except for disclosure to other State cancer registries and local and State health officers" (P.L. 102-515). The regulations must also provide "for a means by which confidential case data may in accordance with State law be disclosed to cancer researchers for the purposes of cancer prevention, control and research."

Almost all of the NPCR programs have established all of the regulations specified in the Cancer Registries Amendment Act on the use of registry information for cancer prevention and control. A number of federal and state approaches to protect privacy of health information (not specific to cancer) are described in Box 5.2.

---

**BOX 5.2  Federal and State Approaches to the Protection of Privacy of Health Information**

**Federal Approaches**

*U.S. Constitution*—While the federal Constitution does not expressly provide individuals with privacy rights, the Supreme Court has recognized a limited right to health informational privacy as a liberty interest within the Fifth and Fourteenth Amendments.

*Federal Statutes*—The federal government has enacted several statutes and regulations to protect privacy of health information:

• **Privacy Act of 1974** requires federal agencies to use fair information practices with regard to the collection, use, or dissemination of systematized records.

- **Freedom of Information Act of 1966 (FOIA)** requires the federal government to provide various information but exempts from governmental disclosure several categories of records which include health information.
- **Electronic Communications Privacy Act of 1986** protects electronic communications during transmission or while in storage against unauthorized interceptions and improper uses, although it likely does not protect interceptions of nonencrypted information over radio frequencies.
- Federal regulations require privacy protections in relation to the administration of human subject research.
- **Health Insurance Portability and Accountability Act (HIPAA)** seeks to reduce the administrative and financial burden of health care by standardizing the electronic transmission of health-related data. HIPAA requires DHHS to set uniform standards for the transmission of health insurance information, including recommendations for security measures to protect private medical information.

The DHHS recommendations focus on five key principles:

1. **Boundaries:** Healthcare information should be disclosed for health purposes only, with limited exceptions.
2. **Security:** Health information should not be distributed unless the patient authorizes it or there is a clear legal basis for doing so. Those who receive such information must safeguard it.
3. **Consumer control:** Persons are entitled to know of and correct information in their health records and the purposes in which it is being used.
4. **Accountability:** Those who improperly hold, distribute, or use health information should be criminally punished, especially when such actions are for monetary gain. Those individuals affected by such actions should have civil recourse.
5. **Public responsibility:** Privacy interests of individuals must not override national priorities of public health, medical research, health services research, healthcare fraud and abuse, and law enforcement in general.

### State Approaches

*State constitutions*—More than a dozen states have adopted constitutional amendments designed to protect a variety of privacy interests, including limitations on access to personal information. Most only protect against breaches of privacy by government.

*State statutes*—States have enacted health information privacy protection in many forms, including laws similar to the federal Privacy Act and FOIA.

*State common law*—State case law imposes duties of confidentiality on certain healthcare professionals not to disclose health information concerning patients.

SOURCE: Hodge, 1999.

Population-based registries have developed a number of policies and procedures to ensure secure handling and processing during data collection, storage, and analysis of confidential data including (NCI, 1999a):

- employees of registries sign pledges to maintain and protect confidential information;
- paper and electronic files are locked in secure areas with restricted access;
- institutional research review committees govern access to confidential information by persons external to the registry;
- written agreements outline the responsibilities of investigators requesting registry data and requirements for maintenance of confidentiality;
- information that could potentially identify an individual, institution, or health-care provider is excluded from public-use data tapes, and analyses of groups are restricted to a sufficiently large size so that personal or institutional identities are obscured; and
- researchers given permission to contact individuals identified in registries must do so through the patient's physician, who seeks permission from the patient to be contacted directly by the researcher.

HIPAA (see description in Box 5.2) requires that national patient identifiers be created, not only for patients, but for employers, providers, and payers. Such identifiers would facilitate data linkages and health services research. The Congress, however, passed a measure that prevents DHHS from using any federal funds to create regulations requiring national patient identifiers, or from assigning numbers (P.L. 105-277, P.L. 106-113; Ziegler, 1999).

In the absence of a unique patient identifier, data linkages currently depend on personal identifiers reported to registries, for example, social security number, name, and birth date. Some individuals do not have social security numbers (e.g., illegal immigrants), and in other cases the social security number may not be available in the medical record (e.g., if not required for reimbursement purposes). Computer programs are available to match records based on all available identifying information (the application of such a program is described in Chapter 4). When personal identifiers are reported to either hospital or state registries, they may be held there and not forwarded to central data repositories. For example, even though NPCR and NCDB require reporting of personal identifying information, the data elements are not forwarded to a central entity at either the CDC or NCDB. The CDC plans to pool state cancer registry data into a Cancer Surveillance System (CSS) to provide national estimates of cancer incidence and to facilitate epidemiologic and health services research. The CDC will not, however, directly receive patient identifiers. It is unclear whether state laws will prohibit the release of confidential data to a third party.[3] Within states,

---

[3]According to the HHS Office for Protection from Research Risks, the NPCR does not need CDC/IRB approval for conducting cancer data collection activities because they

record linkages are often performed by in-house registry staff with Internal Review Board (IRB) approval and are protected by state registry law. While these issues will need to be resolved, there are examples of successful data aggregations and linkages—the NCI has pooled cancer data from its participating registries and linked them to Medicare files while adhering to strict privacy and confidentiality rules (see description of the Medicare-SEER linkage studies in Chapter 4).

## SUMMARY

Relative to the ideal described in Chapter 2, current data systems applicable to cancer care quality assessments have serious shortcomings. No well-established set of quality of care measures exists; consequently, quality assessment initiatives have faced the task of defining such measures for themselves. Quality improvement initiatives have been impeded both by the absence of good cancer care measures and limitations of available data systems. Standards are lacking for reporting factors that are needed in the measurement of the quality of cancer care, for example, stage and comorbidity. Providers do not yet use computer-based patient records, and abstraction of quality information from medical records is time consuming, expensive, and labor intensive. Currently, no data systems are in place with which to make national inferences about the quality of cancer care, and providers do not have benchmarks or targets for gauging their performance relative to others. Despite these shortcomings, there is great potential for enhancing current systems to provide better information on the quality of cancer care.

are considered public health practice surveillance. However, CDC/IRB approval for a call for data through the NPCR-CSS has been applied for and obtained. Such IRB approval is needed because the CSS involves subsequent development of information supplied by NPCR programs into public-use data sets, which could be used for research. In addition to this IRB approval, NPCR has applied for a CDC Assurance of Confidentiality as an extra level of protection for data that will be submitted by NPCR state programs to the CDC (K. Brady, assistant branch chief, NCCDPHP, CDC, personal communication, December 9, 1999).

# 6

# Findings and Recommendations

The National Cancer Policy Board (board) concluded in its April 1999 report, *Ensuring Quality Cancer Care*, that a cancer data system is needed that can provide quality benchmarks for use by systems of care (e.g., hospitals, provider groups, and managed care systems) (IOM, 1999a). Quality assessment studies would ideally include recently diagnosed individuals with cancer in care settings representative of contemporary practice across the country, using information sources with sufficient detail to allow appropriate comparisons. The board recognized that current data systems and quality assessments were far from this ideal.

This chapter summarizes the board's findings and its recommendations for steps that can be taken to enhance current data systems to bring about sustained improvements in cancer care. The board, in its workshop and deliberations, addressed three questions:

1. What would the ideal cancer care data system look like?
2. How are current cancer data systems meeting the needs of healthcare systems?
3. What steps can be taken to enhance data systems so that they can be used to monitor and improve the quality of cancer care?

## WHAT WOULD THE IDEAL CANCER CARE
## DATA SYSTEM LOOK LIKE?

There is no national cancer care data system in the United States. Like the U.S. healthcare system, the data systems available to assess the quality of care on a national or regional basis are fragmented (Pollock, 1997). Advancing quality of care involves applying data in at least three ways:

1. assessing levels and trends in quality of care for whole populations (e.g., the nation, by region, or by state) to identify the magnitude of quality problems and their distribution,
2. determining correlates of quality cancer care (e.g., characteristics of patients and health systems) to elucidate potential causal factors, and
3. measuring and monitoring the quality of cancer care within systems of care to promote quality improvement and allow purchasers and the public to hold systems and providers accountable for the care they deliver.

Health services researchers have creatively exploited available databases to meet these objectives, but most sources can be critiqued on one or more important grounds—a lack of geographic representation or the absence of critical data elements needed to adjust results to make comparisons. The board concluded that to meet national quality-of-care objectives, a cancer care data system (which could include several distinct databases) would have the following 10 attributes:

1. *A set of well-established quality-of care-measures*—a single core set of quality measures must be developed using the best available evidence for the full spectrum of an individual's care—from early detection to palliative and end-of-life care.
2. *Reliance on computer-based patient records for information on patient care and outcomes*—adoption of information technology can improve the timeliness and accuracy of information on the quality of cancer care.
3. *Standard reporting of cancer stage, comorbidity, and processes of care*—national quality assessments depend on the uniform recording of data elements needed to accurately assess care.
4. *National, population-based case selection*—complete ascertainment of incident cancer cases by cancer registries is a prerequisite for national quality assessments, allowing case selection for studies whose results can be generalized to the total population, as well as assessments of quality for important subgroups, for example, individuals of low socioeconomic status, and individuals enrolled in certain types of health plans or delivery systems.
5. *Repeated cross-sectional studies to monitor national trends*—a series of measures is needed to monitor progress over time.

6. *Established benchmarks for quality improvement*—systems of care need information on accepted standards of care (e.g., clinical practice guidelines) with which to measure performance.

7. *Data systems for internal quality assurance purposes*—systems of care need internal data to monitor performance and quality improvement.

8. *Public reporting of selected aggregate quality scores*—quality measures enable consumers and purchasers to judge the quality of a system of care by its performance relative to evidence-based standards.

9. *Adaptability*—new evidence on quality measures, changes in healthcare delivery, and technological innovation are among the factors that necessitate flexibility in data systems.

10. *Protections to ensure privacy of health information*—legal protections and data security systems must be in place to ensure that data collected and stored about an individual's diagnosis and treatment of cancer are used only for legitimate purposes.

## HOW ARE CURRENT CANCER DATA SYSTEMS MEETING THE NEEDS OF HEALTHCARE SYSTEMS?

There are a number of ways for health systems to use available data resources to implement quality improvement programs. Some programs depend entirely on retrospective reviews of medical charts or hospital cancer registry data, while others rely on multiple sources, for example, administrative claims data linked to cancer registry data. Chapter 3 in this report presents 10 case studies to illustrate how various health systems—small physician practices, large integrated delivery systems, professional associations, purchasing coalitions, and states—have used available data to assess cancer care quality (Table 6.1).

The case studies are a testament to creativity—data intended for other purposes have in several instances been manipulated to monitor the quality of care and sometimes appear to have been used within programs to effect improvements in care. The data used by systems of care generally fall into one of the following categories:

• *Retrospective medical chart review*—abstraction of data from medical charts can summarize performance on selected measures of the process or outcomes of care.

• *Cancer registry data*—hospital-based cancer registration programs can provide local data on stage at diagnosis and first course of therapy. In large systems of care, the registry data may be used to identify patients for whom additional clinical information is abstracted from the medical chart.

• *Administrative systems*—billing systems and hospital discharge summaries are sometimes used to assess processes of care for identified populations (sometimes through linkages to cancer registry data).

**TABLE 6.1** Illustrative Case Studies of the Use of Data to Monitor the Quality of Care

| Name (type of organization) | Purpose | Data Source(s) |
| --- | --- | --- |
| 1. Marin Oncology Associates (private oncology practice) | Monitor adherence to guidelines on screening, treatment, follow-up, supportive, and end-of-life care | Medical chart |
| 2. OnCare (Physician Practice Management Company) | Monitor adherence to guidelines on treatment, follow-up, and end-of-life care | Electronic medical chart |
| 3. American College of Radiology | Monitor patterns of care and adherence to guidelines | Medical chart abstraction from a national sample of radiation oncology providers |
| 4. Sutter Health (integrated health care delivery system) | Monitor adherence to breast cancer treatment guidelines | Hospital cancer registry, State cancer registry, administrative data, medical charts, patient surveys |
| 5. Providence Health Plan (integrated delivery system) | Monitor adherence to breast cancer treatment guidelines | Hospital cancer registry, administrative data, medical charts, patient surveys |
| 6. National Comprehensive Cancer Network (17 large cancer centers) | Monitor adherence to breast cancer treatment guidelines | Medical charts. Reporting according to a uniform data set |
| 7. Roswell Park Cancer Institute and private insurers in New York | Monitor adherence to breast cancer treatment guidelines | Insurance claims, medical charts |
| 8. Colorado Cancer Registry, University of Colorado, and the State Medicare Peer Review Organization | Monitor use of adjuvant therapies for breast and colorectal cancer | State cancer registry, Medicare claims, medical charts |
| 9. Central Florida Health Care Coalition (business coalition) | Monitor quality of care for individuals with selected conditions including cancer | Insurance claims, (hospital and outpatient), patient survey |
| 10. National Cancer Data Base (American College of Surgeons, American Cancer Society) | Monitor quality of care for individuals with cancer | Hospital cancer registries, uniform reporting requirements |

- *Patient surveys*—patient satisfaction surveys and surveys to assess the quality of life post treatment may be administered among cancer patients.
- *Uniform data collection*—clinical information systems with data dictionaries and standardized reporting requirements have been put in place to monitor adherence to guidelines.
- *Prospective medical chart review*—computer-based patient records used by a networked group of providers allow the entry and near simultaneous assessment of performance on selected measures of the process or outcomes of care.

The case studies demonstrate several barriers to systematic quality monitoring within healthcare systems:

- *A lack of recognized measures of quality*—each provider group or organization has taken upon itself the task of reviewing evidence, developing guidelines, and identifying measures. These activities are very costly undertakings, require considerable expertise, and need to be continually reviewed in light of new evidence.
- *A heavy reliance on retrospective medical chart reviews to monitor processes of care*—chart abstraction is labor intensive, inefficient, and prone to error relative to the prospective electronic capture of information possible through computer-based patient record systems.
- *An absence of benchmarks with which to measure progress and success*—systems sometimes establish internal benchmarks or practice norms, but there is often no way to compare internal performance to that of other providers. Internal benchmarks may be skewed if certain statistical issues are not taken into account (e.g., providers with small numbers of cases can unduly effect norms).
- *A lack of attention to the full spectrum of cancer care*—for example, the quality of pain management and end-of-life care may be overlooked.

The board did not attempt to survey all cancer-related quality improvement programs but instead wanted to illustrate a variety of approaches. Of note, however, was the difficulty in identifying even 10 initiatives to profile. There do not appear to be many quality improvement programs addressing cancer care, perhaps because of the noted limitations above.

On the other hand, innovations within some of the emerging cancer disease management programs and physician practice management companies are noteworthy. Some have developed sophisticated computer-based patient record systems that prompt physicians with guideline recommendations and system-wide practice norms as they provide care to their patients. Such clinical decision support systems can significantly improve the quality of patient care (Classen, 1998; Hunt, 1998). Data are also captured, stored in a central "data warehouse," and used to monitor adherence to guidelines. The board estimates that approximately 15 to 20% of cancer patients are cared for in environments where these technologies are becoming available (e.g., certain managed care plans and physician practice management companies with computer-based patient record systems [CPRs]) (Mighion, 1999). Medical practice lags behind other industries in applying information technologies, but this may be about to change as new internet-based products targeted to healthcare providers emerge (McDonald, 1998). Significant barriers remain to be overcome before there is widespread adoption of new information technologies in the healthcare sector. Uniform standards, for example, do not yet exist to code and format clinical information within computer-based patient record systems. And even though there are techniques to protect the privacy of electronically stored health information (e.g., encryption, password-driven access), public trust in such technologies is lacking (Goldsmith, 2000).

The absence of a set of recognized measures of cancer care quality is a clear impediment to quality assessment. The development of guidelines through the National Comprehensive Cancer Network (NCCN) seems to have spurred quality monitoring activities beyond the cancer centers that developed them, suggesting that if a core set of cancer care measures were available, it would be adopted by systems of care for quality improvement programs.

Also lacking is a context for measurement. How should health systems focus their quality improvement programs? Should they focus attention on procedures for which there is significant practice variation, consensus guidelines, evidence from randomized clinical trials? A number of patterns-of-care studies have been completed, but with few exceptions, they have not led to vigorous efforts to reduce practice variation. Variation in practice often reflects uncertainty and the lack of good evidence upon which to base treatment decisions. There is, for example, evidence of significant variation in the use of second-, third-, and fourth-line chemotherapy for patients with progressive non-small-cell lung cancer (Smith, 1998). There are no randomized clinical trials comparing best supportive care versus second-line chemotherapy for patients with non-small-cell lung cancer. A guideline could be established based on expert opinion, but guidelines based on sound evidence rather than expert opinion are most likely to succeed in influencing provider practice (OTA, 1994). Priority should be given to implementing measures for which there is practice variation, despite good evidence to support a standard set of practices. For cancer care a few measures would appear to meet this criterion. There is good evidence, for example, to support the use of adjuvant therapy following surgery for breast and colon cancer and evidence of variation in its use (IOM, 1999a).

While quality improvement programs launched within hospitals or integrated health networks are well suited to motivating changes in provider behaviors, population-based studies are necessary to assess progress in quality improvement more broadly. Needed are national or regional studies to:

- assess the extent of quality problems,
- identify correlates of poor quality care,
- establish benchmarks, and

- target interventions to improve care.

At this level, data needs shift. Information is needed for entire populations, not just individuals within certain systems of care. Three well-established data sources for assessing care on a national level are available: the National Program of Cancer Registries (NPCR), the Surveillance, Epidemiology and End Results Program (SEER), and the National Cancer Data Base (NCDB). These three national sources of data on cancer have some common elements. They all, for example, contain hospital-reported cases of cancer, but they differ in most other respects:

- *Purpose*—While NPCR and SEER are focused on surveillance, NCDB is the only system that was actually designed as a tool for monitoring the quality of cancer care. Consequently, NCDB includes more data elements on treatment than either NPCR or SEER.
- *Geographic coverage*—NPCR and NCDB are national in scope, while the SEER registry is limited to a few geographic areas. SEER data are adjusted using population weights to develop national estimates of cancer incidence, but such procedures would not be appropriate in the context of quality-of-care studies because of the unusual distribution of care systems across the country (e.g., managed care penetration, availability of cancer centers). When fully operational, NPCR (together with SEER) has the potential of being a very valuable resource for national cancer care studies because of its near complete geographic coverage.
- *Caseload*—Many fewer cases are processed each year by SEER, and resources are focused on ensuring that the quality of data is high. The completeness, timeliness, and quality of data in the NPCR registries have improved markedly in recent years, but significant variation across states remains.
- *Population-based*—NPCR and SEER are population-based, and rates of cancer can be derived for their respective covered populations. NCDB is largely limited to hospital-reported cases, and certain patients and types of cancer are known to be underrepresented (e.g., patients diagnosed and cared for in outpatient settings). Also, while facilities approved by the American College of Surgeons' Commission on Cancer (ACoS-CoC) are required to report data to NCDB, nonapproved facilities are not, creating a likely bias in ascertainment.

## WHAT STEPS CAN BE TAKEN TO ENHANCE DATA SYSTEMS SO THAT THEY CAN BE USED TO MONITOR AND IMPROVE THE QUALITY OF CANCER CARE?

The board recommends that steps be taken in three areas to enhance data systems to support improvements in the quality of cancer care:

1. Enhance key elements of the data system infrastructure: quality-of-care measures, cancer registries and databases, data collection technologies, and analytic capacity.

2. Expand support for analyses of quality of cancer care using existing data systems.

3. Monitor the effectiveness of data systems to promote quality improvement within health systems.

## 1. Enhance Key Elements of the Data System Infrastructure

*Quality-of-Care Measures*

**Recommendation 1: Develop a single core set of cancer care quality measures.**

Broad consensus has been reached about how to assess some aspects of quality of care for many common cancers, but specific measures are still being developed and tested within health delivery systems. Quality improvement initiatives for cancer care have been impeded both by the absence of thoroughly tested quality measures and limitations of available data systems. The process of developing and testing such measures needs to be stepped up.

As a first step, consensus must be reached on what measures are suitable for immediate use. Major investments in cancer care quality indicators have already been made, but resulting measurement sets have not been widely adopted. The Foundation for Accountability (FAACT), for example, fostered the development of a comprehensive quality indicator set for breast cancer, but few systems of care appear to be using it to assess quality. Barriers to adoption include resistance from plans to new measures, limited resources (e.g., technical assistance), and a lack of technical specifications for adapting measures to different systems of care. Furthermore, given sample size considerations, measures are needed that assess health system competencies across specific diseases, or in the case of cancer, types of cancer (D. Lansky, president, Foundation for Accountability, personal communication, October 13, 1999). There has been a tendency to develop cancer-specific quality measures, but it may be feasible to apply selected measures to all cancer patients or to large segments of patients with cancer. From the board's review of evidence for its report *Ensuring Quality Cancer Care* there appear to be at least some candidate measures that could be broadly applied that merit systematic review (e.g., documentation of cancer stage in medical chart, use of specific recommended adjuvant therapies, appropriate use of palliation, especially pain control).

Since the publication of the board's report, *Ensuring Quality Cancer Care*, some key initiatives have been launched. Both the National Cancer Institute (NCI) and the American Society of Clinical Oncology (ASCO), for example, have taken steps to identify quality-of-care measures (see below). The National

Committee for Quality Assurance (NCQA), an accrediting body for managed care organizations, has designated a medical advisory panel on oncology to identify quality measures. A Department of Health and Human Services (DHHS) committee, the Quality of Cancer Care Committee (QCCC), has been established to focus both on research issues and the delivery of care. The QCCC will work within the structure of the DHHS Quality Improvement Initiative (QII) (NCI, 1999b).

While these disparate efforts are laudable, a coordinated public–private effort is needed to achieve consensus on a single core set of cancer care quality measures. Such measures are needed to assess current practice, target interventions, and to monitor improvements in care.

> **Recommendation 1a: The secretary of the Department of Health and Human Services should designate a committee made up of representatives of public institutions (e.g., the DHHS Quality of Cancer Care Committee, state cancer registries, academic institutions) and private groups (e.g., consumer organizations, professional associations, purchasers, health insurers and plans) to: 1) identify a single core set of quality measures that span the full spectrum of an individual's care and are based on the best available evidence; 2) advise other national groups (e.g., National Committee for Quality Assurance, Joint Commission on the Accreditation of Healthcare Organizations, Quality Forum) to adopt the recommended core set of measures; and 3) monitor the progress of ongoing efforts to improve standard reporting of cancer stage and comorbidity.**

Achieving consensus on a core set of cancer care quality measures may prove to be difficult; however, a number of resources are (or soon will be) available to aid in their identification:

- cancer care guidelines developed by the NCCN,
- the NCI's PDQ (Physician Data Query) system, which provides a summary of evidence related to selected cancer treatments, and
- NCI's forthcoming synthesis of the literature on cancer care outcome measures.

Health services research is needed to test promising quality measures within systems of care, and new research initiatives need to be launched within those areas of cancer care for which there is uncertainty regarding best practices.

> **Recommendation 1b: Research sponsors (e.g., Agency for Healthcare Research and Quality [(AHRQ], National Cancer Institute [NCI], Health Care Financing Administration [HCFA], Depart-**

**ment of Veterans Affairs [VA]) should invest in studies to identify evidence-based quality indicators across the continuum of cancer care.**

Wide variation in clinical practice for certain aspects of cancer care exists, which suggests uncertainty among providers (and to some extent consumers) in the face of alternative treatment options for which there are limited data on effectiveness (e.g., use of surgery for prostate cancer, use of second-, third-, and fourth-line chemotherapy for progressive non-small-cell lung cancer). Clinical trials are usually needed to assess the relative effectiveness of various treatment options. Sometimes, the evidence upon which to make practice recommendations exists but has not been systematically examined. In this case, evidence from the literature may be culled to inform treatment practices. AHRQ's "evidence-based practice centers" (EPCs) provide a mechanism to support such evidence syntheses. The EPCs produce science syntheses that provide the foundation for developing practice guidelines, performance measures, and other quality-related activities. Cancer-related topics to date have included assessments of testosterone suppression treatment of prostatic cancer, and evaluation of cervical cytology (www.ahrq.gov/clinic/epc).

When evidence-based candidate measures are proposed, they need to be tested within healthcare systems. One model for such applied research is the funding from 1996 to 1998 of cooperative agreements as part of "Expanding and Improving Quality of Care Measures" (Q-SPAN). AHRQ and NCQA co-funded Q-SPAN to develop and test clinical performance measures for specific conditions (e.g., cardiovascular diseases, asthma, hip fractures), patient populations, and healthcare settings (www.ahrq.gov/qual/qspanovr.htm). Similarly, HCFA's Diabetes Quality Indicator Project (DQIP) illustrates another successful model for measurement development. Quality indicators were identified and tested through the coordinated efforts of a group of "technical" experts (e.g., clinicians specializing in diabetes care, health services researchers) and an "operations" group made up of representatives of the private sector (e.g., NCQA, FAACT, American Diabetes Association, American Association of Family Physicians, American College of Physicians) and public sector (e.g., HCFA, VA, Centers for Disease Control and Prevention [CDC]). The project benefited from a number of other independent research initiatives (e.g., the Medical Outcomes Study, AHCPR's PORT [Patient Outcomes Research Teams], HCFA's Ambulatory Care Quality Improvement Project) and consequently was able to release a fully tested core quality indicator set in 1998, within 1 year of the project's onset (B. Fleming, Diabetes Quality Indicator Project, HCFA, personal communication, March 24, 2000).

In addition to having general indicators of quality, standardized measures of cancer stage and comorbidity are needed so that apparent differences in quality can be correctly attributed to aspects of health care. Differences in reporting requirements that are burdensome for registrars exist now, but efforts are underway through a collaborative Stage Task Force to standardize data collection for both cancer stage and comorbidity.

**Recommendation 1c: Ongoing efforts to standardize reporting of cancer stage and comorbidity should receive a high priority and be fully supported.**

While first steps to identify and adopt cancer care measures are being taken within the cancer care community, a broadly focused response to quality of healthcare issues is taking shape at the federal level. In the wake of the influential report of the President's Advisory Commission on Consumer Protection and Quality in the Health Care Industry (1998) two complementary bodies have been formed on healthcare quality—one in the public sector to promote interagency coordination among DHHS and other federal agencies (Quality Interagency Coordination Task Force [QuIC]), and the other in the private sector to improve healthcare quality, measurement, and reporting (National Forum for Health Care Quality Measurement and Reporting) (see Chapter 5). The aims and activities of both the QuIC and the Quality Forum are quite relevant to the quality cancer care agenda.

The QuIC's goal is to ensure that all federal agencies involved in purchasing, providing, studying, or regulating healthcare services are working in a coordinated way toward the common goal of improving quality of care. The complementary Quality Forum established with a private-sector base will focus on measurement issues in an effort to ensure system-wide capacity to evaluate and report on the quality of care and to further consumer understanding and use of quality measures.

At the same time, an accountability framework is developing within the private sector that incorporates performance measurement of health plans and other healthcare organizations. Inclusion of cancer care measures into these systems could provide valuable information about cancer care to consumers, purchasers, and providers of care:

- Health plans report quality-of-care data to NCQA, an accrediting body for managed care plans.
- Hospitals and healthcare organizations are surveyed and accredited according to standards established by the JCAHO and since 1997 have been required to participate in a quality performance system.

In summary, a national public–private organizational infrastructure is in place to focus on quality measurement and improvement. At the same time a "system" of accountability has emerged within the private sector.

**Recommendation 1d: Efforts to identify quality of cancer care measures should be coordinated with ongoing national efforts regarding quality of care.**

*Cancer Registries and Databases*

Three national cancer-related databases hold great promise to further quality improvement efforts: NPCR, SEER, and NCDB. NPCR and SEER are cancer surveillance systems with a primary mission of providing population-based estimates with which to understand the occurrence and distribution of cancer. These surveillance systems, however, when linked to other data sources or when used to select individual cases for special studies, have great potential to provide population-based estimates of quality-of-care problems. Although these systems hold promise for such studies, most states do not have the resources to augment their current workload to conduct such studies, which fall outside their primary mission of cancer surveillance. Many states are struggling simply to ensure the basic adequacy of their cancer surveillance systems.

The capacity of states to perform cancer surveillance has been greatly enhanced by NPCR. Since 1994, almost all states have received financial and technical assistance from the CDC, and many have adopted model legislation provided by CDC. With this support the registries' ability to ascertain cases has improved, and many now have achieved at least 90% coverage. Many gaps remain, however, and timeliness of reporting is a problem within many registries. The CDC eventually plans to pool NPCR data centrally and to link the data to other sources, for example, Medicare claims and hospital discharge files. The CDC's first call for data will occur in fiscal year 2000. If completed nationwide (and in collaboration with SEER), this would represent a tremendous opportunity to learn more about the quality of cancer care. Relative to its charge (roughly 1 million cases ascertained per year), the NPCR is rather modestly funded (roughly $24 million in federal funding per year in recent years).

In addition to what can be learned through linkages, special studies could be conducted among a representative sample of individuals with cancer. The databases themselves lack the detailed treatment and comorbidity information needed for most quality-of-care studies. Through special studies, representative samples of patients can be identified through registries and followed up to collect the more detailed standardized comorbidity and treatment data (e.g., by contacting attending physicians by mail or by abstracting records in oncologists' offices).

NPCR and SEER are best suited to providing information through data linkages and as a frame for special studies, either at the level of the state, or ultimately, when state data are pooled, on a national basis. If the NPCR and SEER data were used in these ways, it would not be necessary for registries to add data elements to collection. They would need to be excellent "incident" registries. The CDC and the NCI SEER programs have a tradition of providing assistance to states and could provide technical assistance to states to facilitate linkage and other special studies. The CDC and NCI have recently agreed to increase their level of collaboration in several areas including the sponsorship of registry-related training activities and conduct of research (DHHS, Public Health Service, "Memorandum of Understanding Between the Centers for Disease Control and Prevention and the National Cancer Institute," February 14, 2000, personal communication).

> **Recommendation 2:  Congress should increase support to the CDC for NPCR to improve the capacity of states to achieve complete coverage and timely reporting of incident cancer cases. NPCR's primary purpose is cancer surveillance, but NPCR, together with SEER, has great potential to facilitate national, population-based assessments of the quality of cancer care through linkage studies and by serving as a sample frame for special studies.**

ACoS-CoC and the American Cancer Society (ACS) have long supported the examination of quality of cancer care through the most extensive national data collection effort dedicated to this purpose, NCDB. NCDB has tremendous potential to provide detailed information regarding quality to the approved facilities that report to it (and to the few nonapproved facilities that voluntarily report), thereby encouraging improvements in performance. NCDB is in the process of redesigning its reports to facilities, using a report card format with charts showing facility vs. national norms as benchmarks. Eventually, it may be the case that approval depends in part on performance, or improvement in performance. It is, therefore, an excellent tool for motivating change among providers.

As a source of national information on quality, however, NCDB has limitations because of its lack of complete coverage. This coverage problem may worsen as more and more care shifts to outpatient settings. On the other hand, as care shifts to the ambulatory setting, more such facilities may seek commission approval and report to NCDB. Also, NCDB could become a comprehensive source of cancer care data if facilities treating cancer patients were required by JCAHO or other agencies (e.g., HCFA) to be approved. National estimates of quality care could be derived from NCDB, even with its incomplete coverage, if a sample of nonreporting facilities were identified for supplemental data collection. Weighting techniques could then be used to achieve national estimates.

> **Recommendation 3:  Private cancer-related organizations should join ACS and ACoS to provide financial support for NCDB. Expanded support would facilitate efforts underway to report quality benchmarks and performance data to institutions providing cancer care.**

*Data Collection Technologies*

Some of the first "evidence-based" process measures have taxed available data systems. There are two difficulties as far as quality studies are concerned. First, registries only include information on first treatments, and comprehensive quality studies will depend on data related to the full spectrum of cancer care. Second, it is difficult to gather information on treatment that occurs outside of the reporting facility, and retrieval will only worsen as cancer care increasingly moves into outpatient settings.

The process measure, use of radiation therapy following breast-conserving surgery for breast cancer, illustrates the difficulties. To assess compliance to this standard, a data system must identify women with breast cancer who have undergone breast conserving surgery, and among this group assess the proportion receiving radiation therapy. Registries may be able to identify the "denominator," the number of women who underwent surgery, however, information on subsequent use of radiation therapy may be difficult to obtain, especially if the adjuvant therapy took place outside of the facility reporting the case. The shift of cancer care to outpatient settings has exacerbated reporting problems, and analyses of treatment data from cancer registries show substantial underreporting (Bickell, 2000). Despite the growing difficulties of retrieving treatment data, state registries do not receive any direct financial support for data collection from NPCR or SEER.

ACoS-CoC has quality of cancer care at the core of its mission. Facilities approved by ACoS-CoC have cancer registrars forward to NCDB the same data reported to the state cancer registry along with some additional diagnostic and treatment-related data. NCDB faces the same problem as state cancer registries of limited access to information on subsequent care occurring outside of the reporting facility. In addition, any case diagnosed and treated outside of a hospital could be missed entirely. The burden to facility-based registrars is great, but like NPCR and SEER, NCDB does not currently provide direct support for data collection activities.

How best to collect treatment data for quality-of-care studies needs to be reexamined. Under current systems, state- and facility-based cancer registrars do not have the resources needed to collect complete and accurate treatment data. Perhaps the most effective method of retrieving complete treatment data for quality studies is to link cancer registries to administrative records (e.g., SEER-Medicare, hospitals discharge abstracts) or through special studies. For special studies, registry staff need to have additional resources to gather necessary data.

Alternate funding mechanisms for data reporting for quality purposes have been used by purchasers. Gateway Purchasing Association, a purchasing coalition of businesses in St. Louis, for example, withholds 4% of premiums from the health plans with which it contracts, unless the plan provides the quality information requested by the coalition (e.g., HEDIS® measures). Ultimately, such methods would apply to cancer care if cancer-specific indicators were adopted within HEDIS® or other accepted measurement sets.

**Recommendation 4: Federal research agencies (e.g., NCI, CDC, AHRQ, HCFA) should support research and demonstration projects to identify new mechanisms to organize and finance the collection of data for cancer care quality studies. Current data systems tend to be hospital based, while cancer care is shifting to outpatient settings. New models are needed to capture entire episodes of care, irrespective of the setting of care.**

Advances in information technology will provide many opportunities to improve the quality of cancer care. Clinicians with access to computer-based patient record and Intranet systems, for example, will be better able to:

- uniformly apply stage and comorbidity reporting standards while recording patient data,
- refer to clinical practice guidelines or protocols at the point of care, and
- quickly transmit formatted data to cancer registrars.

There are a few pioneers of such applications among cancer care providers, but adoption of such technologies in health care has lagged behind those of other industries. An Institute of Medicine (IOM) committee charged in 1997 with examining progress toward the development of a CPR concluded that support for CPR research has not been provided in the scope and scale necessary to enable major breakthroughs and that federal funding in the United States has been modest and inconsistent (IOM, 1997).

**Recommendation 5: Federal research agencies (e.g., National Institutes of Health [NIH], Food and Drug Administration [FDA], CDC, VA) should support public–private partnerships to develop technologies, including CPRs and Intranet-based communication systems, that will improve the availability, quality, and timeliness of clinical data relevant to assessing quality of cancer care.**

*Analytic Capacity*

Cancer care data, even when enhanced, are of little use if only a few individuals are trained in their analysis and interpretation. Many methodologic issues need to be resolved in establishing quality improvement systems (e.g., setting benchmarks, creating report card formats for providers and consumers, adjusting for case-mix differences), which will require the concerted efforts of clinicians and health services researchers. Several organizations provide training grants and fellowships (e.g., ACS, Robert Wood Johnson Foundation, NCI, AHRQ), and these should be applied to train investigators in these areas. The creation of "Centers of Excellence" in cancer-related health services research could provide focal points for both training and research.

**Recommendation 6: Federal research agencies (e.g., NCI, AHRQ, VA) should expand support for training in health services research and for training of professionals with expertise in the measurement of quality of care and the implementation and evaluation of interventions designed to improve the quality of care.**

The board reiterates its recommendation made in *Ensuring Quality Cancer Care*, that research sponsors should expand support for cancer-related health services research. In response to the NCPB report, NCI has committed to launching a coordinated program of research to improve the methodological and empirical base for quality-of-care assessment for cancer. As conceived, this research program will evaluate whether observed patterns of care are associated with good outcomes, establish the use of a core set of outcome measures in research and medical care applications, investigate methodologic innovations to improve data collection, and, using the above, promote the development of a national cancer data system to monitor the quality of cancer care (NCI, 1999b). NCI also plans to support cooperative agreements with a consortium of investigator teams that might include one or more of the following: academic institutions, cancer registries, professional associations, cancer centers, and other research organizations (NCI, 1999b).

ASCO is taking the first steps toward the design of a quality monitoring system for cancer patients. In collaboration with RAND/UCLA and Harvard University, ASCO will explore methods to generate timely, reliable, and valid data regarding the quality of cancer care. ASCO will articulate a set of measures of quality cancer care and design a sampling and data collection system that will provide the needed information to assess quality at the level of the provider (ASCO, 2000).

Opportunities for health services research abound with available sources of data. For example, AHRQ's Healthcare Cost and Utilization Project can be used to assess variations in patterns of hospital care and differences in care across systems of care. Only a few cancer-focused health services researchers have analyzed these data. Much more can be learned also from the linked SEER-Medicare database, just updated to include Medicare data through 1998 for persons diagnosed with cancer in 1996. Other recent health services research programs could also provide valuable information related to quality. NCI, for example, has organized a consortium of large managed care plans to promote collaborative research. These health plans have internal information systems and a population-based approach to health care, making them ideal partners for research.

## 2. Expand Support for Analyses of Quality of Cancer Care Using Existing Data Systems.

One issue under debate is whether cancer registries, with their primary mission of cancer surveillance, should be augmented to meet the needs of quality assessment, or whether an entirely new system needs be designed, tailored to the needs of quality assessment. One single, integrated database probably cannot meet all of the various objectives of such systems, for example, cancer surveillance, research, and quality monitoring. Such a system would be complex, cumbersome, and terribly costly. Despite some shortcomings, available data systems have been used in creative ways through linkages and as sampling frames for in-depth special studies. With enhancements of elements of current systems, these approaches, if widely applied, could answer many outstanding questions about the quality of cancer care, on a national scale, and without delays of many years between data collection and analysis.

One of the most productive strategies researchers have used to assess the quality of cancer care has been to link cancer registry data to either administrative records or hospital discharge files. The data sources are often complementary—cancer registry data have good information on diagnosis and cancer stage but may not record complete information on treatment. Administrative data may lack the diagnostic information but have a good record of treatment encounters. The linkage approach is not without problems. Administrative records may have treatments miscoded, comorbidity data needed to adjust results may be limited, and data elements necessary for complete linkage may be absent. Nevertheless, such linkages have allowed researchers to study variation in cancer care and to make comparisons across systems of care. In one notable example, the appropriateness of treatment of elderly Colorado residents with breast or colon cancer was assessed through a linkage between the cancer registry and the Medicare claims files. Following the finding of significant underuse of adjuvant therapy among older patients (verified by chart review and controlling for comorbidity), an extensive educational campaign was launched to address the problem. This project was undertaken in collaboration with the state Peer Review Organization (PRO). Each state has a PRO funded by HCFA, which evaluates whether care given to Medicare patients is reasonable, necessary, and provided in the most appropriate setting. The most recent contract with HCFA (totaling more than $1 billion) requires PROs to conduct local quality improvement projects on six clinical prioritized areas, one of which is breast cancer (Jencks, 1999). The board recommends that PROs across the country use the Colorado linkage study as a model as they plan their quality improvement initiatives.

Many cancer registries are achieving near complete levels of case ascertainment, making them valuable as sampling frames for targeted special studies. Here, cancer registry staff may be asked to gather from medical charts, or contacts with reporting physicians, clinical information to supplement that obtained for registry purposes. With appropriate resources, special studies can be launched relatively quickly in response to specific research questions. Some state laws regarding confidentiality and consent have made timely access to research subjects difficult (e.g., requiring consent from patients and the attending physician); however, this approach provides an efficient mechanism to identify and then conduct follow-up among selected patients.

**Recommendation 7: Federal research agencies (e.g., NCI, AHRQ, VA) should expand support for health services research, especially studies based on the linkage of cancer registry to administrative data and special studies of cases sampled from cancer registries. Resources should also be made available through the NPCR and SEER programs to provide technical assistance to states to help them expand the capability of using cancer registry data for quality improvement initiatives. NPCR should also be supported in its efforts to consolidate state data and link them to national data files.**

Other opportunities to evaluate cancer care regionally occur without reliance on cancer registry data. For example, a group of private insurers has joined researchers at Roswell Park Cancer Institute to evaluate the quality of care among their covered population using insurance claims data. Coalitions of businesses have also formed to evaluate the quality of care using their pooled claims data. The board applauds efforts by private insurers and employers to measure and improve the quality of cancer within their respective populations.

Much can be learned about the quality of cancer care by linking data from cancer registries to other sources, such as insurance records. Questions arise, however, regarding who should have access to the personal identifying information needed to conduct such linkages, and whether the individual identities of patients recorded in electronic databases can be held in confidence. No legal action regarding a breach of confidentiality from cancer registries or other databases is known to have occurred in the United States, but the potential for a breach necessitates that adequate safeguards be in place. Recent federal legislation (the Health Insurance Portability and Accountability Act) established legal sanctions for wrongful disclosure of individually identifiable health information and called for the secretary of Health and Human Services to provide detailed recommendations on privacy of health data and procedures and rules for authorized disclosure of such information (IOM, 1997).

As the quality of state cancer registries improves and as efforts to link registry data to other sources proceed, either at the state or national level, models should be developed for how such linkages should be conducted, and how resulting databases can be released to researchers without compromising the identification of patients or providers. Nontechnical approaches to protecting privacy include: limiting researcher access to the data (e.g., requiring a formal application for use), having signed agreements to confidentiality rules, and forbidding publication of analyses at low levels of geography or for very small groups (e.g., rare cancers). NCI follows these and other procedures when releasing to health services researchers data from the SEER-Medicare linked files. The National Center for Health Statistics (NCHS) has established a data center where researchers wishing to link proprietary or other data to national survey data may do so under very controlled conditions (www.cdc.gov/nchs/r&d/rdc.htm). Technical approaches to protecting electronic health information include authentication (e.g., use of IDs and passwords), audit trails (i.e., electronic tracking of access events), and encryption (e.g., limiting access of data to those with an encryption key to decode data) (NRC, 1997). In accordance with the Health Insurance Portability and Accountability Act, DHHS has developed rules setting standards assuring that individual systems have adequate security and an organizational policy to protect data security (Hodge, 1999; Hodge et al., 1999; Ziegler, 1999).

> **Recommendation 8: Federal research agencies (e.g., NCI, AHRQ, HCFA) should develop models for the conduct of linkage studies and the release of confidential data for research purposes that protect the confidentiality and privacy of healthcare information.**

### 3. Monitor the Effectiveness of Data Systems to Promote Quality Improvement Within Health Systems.

Ideally, investments in data systems contribute to quality improvement within health systems. Theory would suggest that quality within health systems improves when organizations measure and monitor performance, encourage change through incentive systems and education, and hold providers accountable to the quality expectations of purchasers and consumers. This market-driven approach to quality improvement holds promise, but there are relatively few examples of full implementation and successful outcomes to motivate its widespread adoption. Evidence of the success of data-driven quality improvement initiatives are needed for cancer care.

> **Recommendation 9: Federal research agencies (e.g., NCI, AHRQ, HCFA, VA) should fund demonstration projects to assess the application of quality monitoring programs within healthcare systems and the impact of data-driven changes in the delivery of services on the quality of health care. Findings from the demonstrations should be disseminated widely to consumers, payers, purchasers, and cancer care providers.**

In summary, the broad availability of cancer-specific data resources makes cancer a unique disease for targeting quality improvement initiatives in patient care. The board is confident that, with a concerted effort, these resources could provide invaluable insights into the quality of contemporary cancer care and point the way to improved care.

# References

Adams-Cameron M, Gilliland FD, Hunt WC, et al. 1999. Trends in incidence and treatment for ductal carcinoma in situ in Hispanic, American Indian, and non-Hispanic white women in New Mexico, 1973–1994. *Cancer* 85(5):1084–1090.

Agency for Healthcare Research and Quality (AHRQ). 2000. Healthcare Cost and Utilization Project (HCUP). http://www.ahcpr.gov/data/hcup.

Agency for Healthcare Research and Quality (AHRQ). 2000. Evidence-Based Practice Centers (EPCs). http://www.ahcpr.gov/clinic/epc/.

Agency for Healthcare Research and Quality (AHRQ). 1999. Expanding and Improving Quality of Care Measures (Q-SPAN). http://www.ahcpr.gov/qual/qspanovr.htm.

Agency for Healthcare Research and Quality (AHRQ). 1997. Theory and Reality of Value-Based Purchasing: Lessons from the Pioneers (AHCPR Pub. No. 98-0004). http://www.ahcpr.gov/qual/meyerrpt.htm.

Aldrich TE, Vann D, Moorman PG, et al. 1995. Rapid reporting of cancer incidence in a population-based study of breast cancer: One constructive use of a central cancer registry. *Breast Cancer Res Treat* 35:61–64.

Allison J, Kiefe CI, Weissman NW. 1999. Can data-driven benchmarks be used to set the goals for Healthy People 2010? *Am J Pub Health* 89:61–65.

American Cancer Society. 1998. *Cancer Facts and Figures—1998*. Atlanta, GA: American Cancer Society.

American Medical Association (AMA). "AMA Study Finds that Physician Web Use Has Doubled." Press release: December 6, 1999. http://www.ama-assn.org/ad-com/releases/1999/991203b.htm.

AMA, American Medical Accreditation Program (AMAP). 1999. http://www.ama-assn.org/med-sci/amapsite.

AMA, AMAP. 1999. AMAP Criteria for AMAP-Compatible Physician Performance Measurement Systems. May 25.

American Society for Clinical Oncology (ASCO). "First Large-Scale Study on Quality Cancer Care Launched." Press release: January 20, 2000. http://www.asco.org/people/nr/html/genpr/m_0100qualitypr.htm.

Austin DF. 1994. Types of Registries: Goals and Objectives. In Menck H and Smart CR, eds. *Central Cancer Registries: Design, Management, and Use.* Amsterdam: Harwood Academic Publishers.

Ayanian JZ. 1999. Using Cancer Registries to Assess Quality of Cancer Care. Presentation at National Cancer Policy Board Workshop, "Enhancing Data Systems to Improve the Quality of Cancer Care," Washington, DC, October 4.

Ayanian JZ, Kohler BA, Abe T, et al. 1993. The relation between health insurance coverge and clinical outcomes among women with breast cancer. *N Engl J Med* 329(5):326–331.

Baker F. 1999. Data for Health Services Research: American Cancer Society, Cancer Survivorship Surveys. Presentation at National Cancer Policy Board Workshop, "Enhancing Data Systems to Improve the Quality of Cancer Care," Washington, DC, October 5.

Ballard DJ. 1999. A call to action: Improving oncologic care information in the United States. *Med Care* 37(5):431–433.

Bergmann MV, Calle EE, Mervis CA, et al. 1998. Validity of self-reported cancers in a prospective cohort study in comparison with data from state cancer registries. *Am J Epidemiol* 147:556–562.

Bickell NA and Chassin MR. 2000. Determining the quality of breast cancer care: Do tumor registries measure up? *Ann Int Med* 132:705–710.

Bland KI, Menck HR, Scott-Conner CE, et al. 1998. The National Cancer Data Base 10-Year survey of breast carcinoma treatment at hospitals in the United States. *Cancer* 83(6):1262–1273.

Bodenheimer T. 1999. The American health care system: The movement for improved quality in health care. *N Engl J Med* 340(6):488–492.

Brown M. 1999. Data for Health Services Research: NCI's HMO Cancer Research Network. Presentation at National Cancer Policy Board Workshop, "Enhancing Data Systems to Improve the Quality of Cancer Care," Washington, DC, October 4.

Castles AG, Milstein A, Damberg CL. 1999. Using employer purchasing power to improve the quality of perinatal care. *Pediatrics* 103(1 Suppl E):248–254.

Chambers LW, Spitzer WO, Hill GB, et al. 1976. Underreporting of cancer in medical surveys: A source of systematic error in cancer research. *Am J Epidemiol* 104(2): 141–145.

Chen VW and Rainey JM. 1996. Louisiana Tumor Registry: New developments and services provided. *J La State Med Soc* 148:186–188.

Chen VW, Wu XC, Andrews PA, eds. 1999. *Cancer in North America: 1991–1995. Volume 1: Incidence.* Sacramento, CA: North American Association of Central Cancer Registries.

Cherney BJ. 1999. President/CEO, Central Florida Health Care Coalition. Personal communication to M. Hewitt, November 23.

Classen DC. 1998. Clinical decision support systems to improve clinical practice and quality of care. *JAMA* 280(15):1360–1361.

Clive RE, Ocwieja KM, Kamell L, et al. 1995. A national quality improvement effort: Cancer registry data. *J Surg Oncol* 58:155–161.

Coia LR, Owen JB, Hanks GE. 1997. Introduction. *Sem Radiat Oncol* 7 (2)3:95–96.

Coleman MP, Muir CS, Menogoz F. 1992. Confidentiality in the cancer registry. *Br J Cancer* 66:1138–1149.

Crane, 1999. Accreditation Programs for Physicians, AMA's AMAP Program. Presentation at National Cancer Policy Board Workshop, "Enhancing Data Systems to Improve the Quality of Cancer Care," Washington, DC, October 4.

Darby M. 1998. Health care quality: From data to accountability. *Acad Med* 73(8):843–853.

Deleyiannis FW, Weymuller EA, Garcia I, et al. 1997. Geographic variation in the utilization of esophagoscopy and bronchoscopy in health and neck cancer. *Arch Otolaryngol Head Neck Surg* 123:1203–1210.

Department of Health and Human Services (DHHS), Centers for Disease Control and Prevention. National Center for Health Statistics. 1999. http://www.cdc.gov/nchs.

DHHS, Centers for Disease Control and Prevention (CDC). 2000. The National Program of Cancer Registries. Cancer Registries: The Foundation for Comprehensive Cancer Control, at a Glance 2000. http://www.cdc.gov/cancer/ncpr/register.htm.

DHHS, Centers for Disease Control and Prevention. 1999. National Program of Cancer Registries Cancer Surveillance System (NPCR-CSS): Rationale and Approach.

DHHS, Centers for Disease Control and Prevention, National Center for Health Statistics. 1999. Research Data Center. http://www/cdc.gov.nchs.r&d.rdc.htm.

DHHS, Office of Public Health and Science, Office of Disease Prevention and Health Promotion. 1996. *Guide to Clinical Preventive Services, Second Edition, Report of the U.S. Preventive Services Task Force.* Washington, DC: DHHS.

DHHS, Centers for Disease Control and Prevention. 1998. Cancer Objectives (Number 15): Statewide Population-Based Cancer Registries. *Healthy People 2010 Objectives: Draft for Public Comment.* Atlanta, GA: CDC.

Desch CE, Penberthy L, Newschaffer CJ, et al. 1996. Factors that determine the treatment for local and regional prostate cancer. *Med Care* 34(2):152–162.

Du X, Freeman JL, Goodwin JS. 1999. Information on radiation treatment in patients with breast cancer: the advantages of the linked Medicare and SEER data. *J Clin Epidemiol* 52(5):463–470.

Eddy DM. 1997. Performance measurement: Problems and solutions. *Health Affairs (Millwood)* 17(4):7–25.

Edge SB, Fritz A, Clutter GG, et al. 1999. A unified cancer stage data collection system: Preliminary report from the Collaborative Stage Task Force/American Joint Committee on Cancer. *J Registry Manage* 26(2):57–61.

Edwards BK. 1997. Associate director, Cancer Surveillance Research Program, Division of Cancer Control and Population Sciences, National Cancer Institute. National Cancer Institute Cancer Surveillance Research. Presentation to the National Cancer Policy Board, July 17.

Fleming St, Kohrs FP. 1998. Linking claims and cancer registry data: Is it worth the effort? *Clin Perform Qual Health Care* 6(2):88–96.

Foundation for Accountability (FACCT). 1998. FACCT Quality Measures—Breast Cancer. http://www.facct.org.

Frey CM, McMillen MM, Cowan CD, et al. 1992. Representativeness of the Surveillance, Epidemiology, and End Results Program data: Recent trends in cancer mortality rates. *J Natl Cancer Inst* 84(11):872–877.

Goldsmith J. 2000. How will the internet change our health system? *Health Affairs* 19(1):148–156.

Greenfield S, Aronow HU, Elashoff RM, et al. 1988. Flaws in mortality data: The hazards of ignoring comorbid disease. *JAMA* 260(15):2253–2255.

Hand R, Sener S, Imperato J, et al. 1991. Hospital variables associated with quality of care for breast cancer patients. *JAMA* 226 (24):3429–3432.

Hanks GE, Coia LR, Curry J. 1997. Patterns of Care studies: Past, present, and future. *Sem Radiat Oncol* 7(2):97–100.

Healthcare Information and Management Systems Society (HIMSS). 1999. 10th Annual HIMSS Leadership Survey Sponsored by IBM: Trends in Healthcare Information and Technology—Final Report. http://www.himss.org/survey.

The Henry J. Kaiser Family Foundation. 1999. *Medicare State Profiles: State and Regional Data on Medicare and the Population It Serves.* Menlo Park, CA: The Henry J. Kaiser Family Foundation.

Hillner B, Penberthy L, Desch CE, et al. 1996. Variation in staging and treatment of local and regional breast cancer in the elderly. *Breast Cancer Res Treat* 40:75–86.

Hillner BE, McDonald MK, Penberthy L, et al. 1997. Measuring standards of care for early breast cancer in an insured population. *J Clin Oncol* 15(4):1401–1408.

Hodge JG. 1999. Privacy Issues Related to Using Registry Data to Monitor Quality of Care. Presentation at National Cancer Policy Board Workshop, "Enhancing Data Systems to Improve the Quality of Cancer Care," Washington, DC, October 4.

Hodge JG, Gostin LO, Jacobson PD. 1999. Legal issues concerning electronic health information: Privacy, quality, and liability. *JAMA* 282(15):1466–1471.

Howe HL, Population-Based Cancer Registries in the United States. Undated manuscript.

Howe HL, Katterhagen JG, Yates J, et al. 1992. Urban–rural differences in the management of breast cancer. *Cancer Causes Control* 3:533–539.

Hunt DL, Haynes RB, Hanna SE, et al. 1998. Effects of computer-based clinical decision support systems on physician performance and patient outcomes: A systematic review. *JAMA* 280(15):1339–1346.

IMSystem. 1997. *Oncology Indicators: Indicator Information Forms, Code Tables, Report Prototype.* Oakbrok Terrace, IL: Joint Commission on Accreditation of Healthcare Organizations.

Institute of Medicine (IOM). 1997. *The Computer-Based Patient Record: An Essential Technology for Health Care* (revised edition). Washington, DC: National Academy Press.

Institute of Medicine. 1999a. *Ensuring the Quality of Cancer Care.* Washington, DC: National Academy Press.

Institute of Medicine. 1999b. *Measuring the Quality of Health Care.* Washington, DC: National Academy Press.

Institute of Medicine. 1999c. *Using Information Technology to Improve Quality in Health Care: Workshop Summary.* Washington DC: Institute of Medicine.

Jencks S. 1999. HCFA's Use of Cancer Care Qualty Data. Presentation at National Cancer Policy Board Workshop, "Enhancing Data Systems to Improve the Quality of Cancer Care," Washington, DC, October 4.

Jessup JM, Menck HR, Winchester DP, et al. 1996. The National Cancer Data Base report on patterns of hospital reporting. *Cancer* 78(8):1829–1837.

Johantgen ME, Coffey RM, Harris DR, et al. 1995. Treating early-stage breast cancer: Hospital characteristics associated with breast-conserving surgery. *Am J Public Health* 85(10):1432–1434.

Johnson CH, ed. 1999. *Standards for Cancer Registries, Volume II. (Data Standards and Data Dictionary* (4th ed). Sacramento, CA: North American Association of Centralized Cancer Registries.

Joint Commission on the Accreditation of Health Care Organizations. 1999. http://www.jcaho.org

Karagas MR, Thomas DB, and Roth GJ. 1991. The effects of changes in health care delivery on the reported incidence of cutaneous melanoma in western Washington State. *Am J Epidemiol* 133:58–62.

Katterhagen G. 1999. Implementing successful internal quality monitoring: Sutter Breast Health Project. Presentation at National Cancer Policy Board Workshop, "Enhancing Data Systems to Improve the Quality of Cancer Care." Washington, DC, October 5.

Katz SJ, Hislop G, Thomas DB, et al. 1993. Delay from symptom to diagnosis and treatment of breast cancer in Washington State and British Columbia. *Med Care* 31(3):264–268.

Kiefe CI, Weissman NW, Allison JJ, et al. 1998. Identifying achievable benchmarks of care: Concepts and methodology. *Int J Qual Health Care* 10(5):443–447.

KnowMed. 1999. http://www.knowmed.com.

Koh HK, Clapp RW, and Barnett JM. 1991. Systemic underreporting of cutaneous malignant melanoma in Massachusetts. *J Am Acad Dermatol* 24:545–550.

Kurowski B. 1996. Cancer carve outs and outcomes measurement programs: An emerging paradigm. *Med Interface* 9(11):81–84.

Lazar GS and Desch CE. 1998. Performance measurement in cancer care: Uses and challenges. *Cancer* 82(Suppl 10):2016–2021.

Lieberman MD, Kilburn H, Lindsey M, et al. 1995. Relation of perioperative deaths to hospital volume among patients undergoing pancreatic resection for malignancy. *Ann Surg* 222(5):638–645.

Lu-Yao GL, Greenberg ER. 1994. Changes in prostate cancer incidence and treatment in USA. *Lancet* 343:251–254.

Lu-Yao GL, Potosky AL, Albertsen, et al. 1996. Follow-up prostate cancer treatments after radical prostatectomy: A population-based study. *J Natl Cancer Inst* 88(3/4): 166–173.

Malin JL, Asch SM, Kerr EA, and McGlynn EA. 2000. Evaluating the quality of cancer care: Development of cancer quality indicators for a global quality assessment tool. *Cancer* 88(3)701–707.

Mandelblatt JS, Ganz PA, Kahn KL. 1999. Proposed agenda for the measurement of quality of care outcomes in oncology practice. *J Clin Oncol* 17(8):2614–2622.

Mann BA, Samet JM, Hunt WC, et al. 1988. Changing treatment of breast cancer in New Mexico from 1969 through 1985. *JAMA* 259(23):3413–3417.

McDonald CJ, Overhage JM, Dexter PR, et al. 1998. Canopy computing: Using the Web in clinical practice. *JAMA* 280(15):1325–1329.

McGlynn E. 1998. Choosing and evaluating clinical performance measures. *Joint Comm J Qual Improve* 24:470–479.

Menck HR, Bland KI, Conner CEH, et al. 1998. Regional diversity and breadth of the National Cancer Data Base. *Cancer* 83(12):2649–2658.

Menck HR, Cunningham MP, Jessup JM, et al. 1997. The growth and maturation of the National Cancer Data Base. *Cancer* 80(12):2296–2306.

Mighion K, Gesme, DH, Rifkin RM, et al. 1999. Growth of oncology physician management companies. *Cancer Invest* 17(5):362–370.

Miller A. 1999. Involving physicians in cancer disease management: Ten concepts. *Managed Care Cancer* 1(6):26–30.

*Modern Healthcare's "By the Numbers."* 1999. HMO Market Penetration by State: Interstudy. July 19.

Morris D. Data for Health Services Research: AHCPR, Healthcare Cost and Utilization Project. Presentation at National Cancer Policy Board Workshop, "Enhancing Data Systems to Improve the Quality of Cancer Care," Washington, DC, October 5.

Morrow M. 1999. Using hospital-based data to monitor physicians and hospitals: The National Cancer Data Base. Presentation at National Cancer Policy Board Workshop, "Enhancing Data Systems to Improve the Quality of Cancer Care," Washington, DC, October 4.

Moulton G. 1998. Database provides window on applications of treatments. *J Natl Cancer Inst* 90(24):1865–1866.

Munoz KA, Harlan LC, Trimble EL. 1997. Patterns of care for women with ovarian cancer in the United States. *J Clin Oncol* 15(11):3408–3415.

National Cancer Institute (NCI). 2000. NCI and CDC Collaborate on a Comprehensive Cancer Surveillance and Control System. Press release: March 17. http://rex.nci.nih.gov/massmedia/pressreleases.nci_cdc.html.

NCI. 1999a. Confidentiality, Data Security, and Cancer Research: Perspectives from the NCI. www.nci.nih.gov/confidentiality.html.

NCI. 1999b. Response to *Ensuring Quality Care*, a Report of the National Cancer Policy Board. Unpublished.

NCI, Surveillance Implementation Group (SIG). 1999. *Cancer Surveillance Research Implementation Plan*. Bethesda, MD: NCI.

National Committee for Quality Assurance. 1999. http://www.ncqa.org.

National Comprehensive Cancer Network. 1999. Member Institutions. http://www.nccn.org/network_content.htm.

National Quality Forum. 2000. Mission Statement. http://www.qualityforum.org/mission/.

National Research Council. 1997. *For the Record: Protecting Electronic Health Information*. Washington, DC: National Academy Press.

Nattinger AB, Hoffmann RG, Shapiro R, et al. 1996. Effect of legislative requirements on the use of breast-conserving surgery. *N Engl J Med* 335(14):1035–1040.

Nattinger AB, McAuliffe TL, Schapira MM. 1997. Generalizability of the Surveillance, Epidemiology, and End Results Registry population: Factors relevant to epidemiologic and health care research. *J Clin Epidemiol* 50(8):939–945.

Newcombe HB. 1995. When "privacy" threatens public health. *Can J Public Health* 86(3):188–192.

Newcomer LN. 1997. Keynote address: Deodorants, value and performance. *NCCN Proc* 11:21–24.

North American Association of Central Cancer Registries. 1999. Mission, goals, and objectives 1996–2000. http://www.naaccr.org.

O'Kane ME. 2000. President, National Committee for Quality Assurance. Presentation to the Committee on the National Quality Report on Health Care Delivery, Institute of Medicine, Washington, DC, February 14.

Office of Management and Budget. 2000. Statistical programs of the United States government: Fiscal Year 2000. Washington, DC: Office of Management and Budget.

OnCare. 1998. http://www. oncare.com.

Oncology News. 1999. NCQA to add more measures of the quality of cancer care to its HEDIS performance dataset. *Oncol News* 8(4):2, 20.

Partridge EE. 1998. The National Cancer Data Base: Ten years of growth and commitment. *CA Cancer J Clin* 48(3):131–145.

Penman AD, Brackin BT, and Moulder JT. 1996. Case report: Mississippi's new central cancer registry design and implementation. *J Miss State Med Assoc* 37(4):537–539.

Piccirillo JF. 1999. Data Elements Needed for Quality Assessment. Presentation at National Cancer Policy Board Workshop, "Enhancing Data Systems to Improve the Quality of Cancer Care," Washington, DC, October 4.

Piccirillo JF, Creech C, Zequeira R, et al. 1999. Inclusion of comorbidity into oncology data registries. *J Registry Manage* 26(2):66–70.

Polednak AP. 1997. Predictors of breast-conserving surgery in Connecticut, 1990–1992. *Ann Surg Oncol* 4(3):259–263.

Polednak AP, Shevchenko IP, Flannery JT, et al. 1996. Estimating breast cancer treatment charges in Connecticut. *Conn Med* 60(5)263–267.

Polednak AP and Flannery JT. 1992. Black versus white racial differences in clinical stage at diagnosis and treatment of prostatic cancer in Connecticut. *Cancer* 70(8): 2152–2158.

Pollock AM, Rice DP. 1997. Monitoring health care in the United States: A challenging task. *Public Health Rep* 112:109–115.

Potosky AL. 1999. Using SEER to Answer Quality-Related Health Services Research. Presentation at National Cancer Policy Board Workshop, "Enhancing Data Systems to Improve the Quality of Cancer Care," Washington, DC, October 4.

Potosky AL, Harlan LC, Stanford JL, et al. 1999. Prostate cancer practice patterns and quality of life: The Prostate Cancer Outcomes Study. *J Natl Cancer Inst* 91(20): 1719–1724.

Potosky AL, Riley GF, Lubitz J, et al. 1993. Potential for cancer related health services research using a linked Medicare-tumor registry database. *Med Care* 31(8):732–748.

Potosky AL, Merrill RM, Riley GF, et al. 1997. Breast cancer survival and treatment in health maintenance organization and fee-for-service settings. *J Natl Cancer Inst* 89(22):1683–1691.

Potosky AL, Merrill RM, Riley GF, et al. 1999. Prostate cancer treatment and 10-year survival among group/staff HMO and fee-for-service Medicare patients. *Health Serv Res* 34(2):525–546.

President's Advisory Commission. 1999. *Consumer Protection and Quality in the Health Care Industry, Final Report.* http://www.hcqualitycommission.gov/final/.

Public Law 102-515. *Cancer Registries Amendment Act.* October 24, 1992.

Public Law 105-277. *FY1999 Omnibus Appropriations Act.* October 21, 1999.

Public Law 106-113. *DHHS Appropriation Act for FY2000.* November 1999.

Quality Interagency Coordination Task Force. 2000. Agency for Healthcare Research and Quality Fact Sheet. http://www.ahcpr.gov/qual/quicfact.htm.

Quality Oncology, Inc. 1999. Brochure and Fact Sheet. McLean, VA: Quality Oncology, Inc.

Riley GF, Feuer EJ, et al. 1996. Disenrollment of Medicare cancer patients from health maintenance organizations. *Med Care* 34(8):826–836.

Riley GF, Potosky AL, Klabunde CN, et al. 1999. Stage at diagnosis and treatment patterns among older women with breast cancer. *JAMA* 281(8):720–726.

Roohan PJ, Bickell NA, Baptiste MS, et al. 1998. Hospital volume difference and five-year survival from breast cancer. *Am J Public Health* 88(3):454–457.

Salick Health Care, Inc. 1999. www.salick.com.

Schuster MA, Reifel JL, McGuigan K. 1998a. Assessment of the Quality of Cancer Care. Paper prepared for the National Cancer Policy Board, Washington, DC.

Schuster MA, McGlynn EA, Brook RH. 1998b. How good is the quality of health care in the United States? *Milbank Q* 76(4):517–563.

Sener SF, Fremgen A, Menck HR, et al. 1999. Pancreatic cancer: A report of treatment and survival trends for 100,313 patients diagnosed from 1985–1995, using the National Cancer Database. *J Am Coll Surgeons* 89(1):1–7.

Sennett C. 1999. A glimpse at the National Committee for Quality Assurance. *Managed Care Cancer* May/June:40–41.

Smith TJ, Hillner NE. 1998. Ensuring Quality Cancer Care: Clinical Practice Guidelines, Critical Pathways, and Care Maps. Paper prepared for the National Cancer Policy Board, Washington, DC.

Smith TJ, Penberthy L, Desch CE, et al. 1995. Differences in initial treatment patterns and outcomes of lung cancer in the elderly. *Lung Cancer* 13:235–252.

Swan J, Wingo P, Clive R, et al. 1998. Cancer surveillance in the U.S.: Can we have a national system? *Cancer* 83(7):1282–1291.

Tucker TC, Howe HL, and Weir HK. 1999. Certification for population-based registries. *J Registry Manage* Feb:24–27.

U.S. Congress, Office of Technology Assessment. 1994. Identifying Health Technologies that Work: Searching for Evidence. Washington, DC: U.S. GPO.

Wagner G. 1991. History of Cancer Registration. In Jensen OM, Parkin DM, MacLennan R, et al., eds. *Cancer Registration: Principles and Methods*. Lyons, France: International Agency for Research on Cancer.

Wanebo HJ, Cole B, Chung M, et al. 1997. Is surgical management compromised in elderly patients with breast cancer? *Ann Surg* 225(5):579–589.

Warren J, Potosky A, and Riley J. 1999. Use of linked SEER-Medicare Data: Assessing Quality of Care. Presentation at National Cancer Policy Board Workshop, "Enhancing Data Systems to Improve the Quality of Cancer Care," Washington DC, October 4.

Watkins S, MacKinnon J, W Price. 1994. Legislation, Affiliation and Governance. In Menck H and Smart C, eds. *Central Cancer Registries: Design, Management, and Use*. Amsterdam: Harwood Academic Publishers.

Weeks JC. 1997. Outcomes assessment in the NCCN. *NCCN Proc* 11:137–140.

Weeks JC. 1999. National Comprehensive Cancer Network. Presentation at National Cancer Policy Board Workshop, "Enhancing Data Systems to Improve the Quality of Cancer Care," Washington, DC, October 4.

Weeks JC and Niland JC. 1999. NCCN oncology outcomes database: An update. *Managed Care Cancer* May/June:32–35.

Weissman NW, Allison JJ, Kiefe CI et al. 1999. Achievable benchmarks of care: The ABCs of benchmarking. *J Eval Clin Pract* 5(3):269–281.

Wingo P. 1999. Data for health services research: National Center for Health Statistics, National Hospital Discharge Survey. Presentation at National Cancer Policy Board Workshop, "Enhancing Data Systems to Improve the Quality of Cancer Care," Washington, DC, October 5.

Winn R. 1999. Accreditation programs for health plans: National Committee for Quality Assurance. Presentation at National Cancer Policy Board Workshop, "Enhancing Data Systems to Improve the Quality of Cancer Care," Washington, DC, October 4.

Ziegler J. 1999. Inching toward an info technology revolution. In "The State of Healthcare in America." *Business and Health* 15(5, Suppl A):50–55.

# Acronyms and Abbreviations

| | |
|---|---|
| ABC™ | achievable benchmarks of care |
| ACoS-CoC | American College of Surgeons' Commission on Cancer |
| ACR | American College of Radiology |
| ACS | American Cancer Society |
| AHRQ | Agency for Healthcare Research and Quality |
| AJCC | American Joint Committee on Cancer |
| AMI | acute myocardial infarction |
| ASCO | American Society of Clinical Oncology |
| | |
| BCS | breast conserving surgery |
| | |
| CAHPS | Consumer Assessment of Health Plans Survey |
| CARES | Cancer Rehabilitation Evaluation System |
| CDC | Centers for Disease Control and Prevention |
| CFHCC | Central Florida Health Care Coalition |
| CPR | computer-based patient record |
| CRN | Cancer Research Network |
| CSS | Cancer Surveillance System |
| | |
| DCS | ductal carcinoma in situ |
| DHHS | Department of Health and Human Services |
| DQIP | Diabetes Quality Indicator Project |
| DRGs | diagnosis related groups |

| | |
|---|---|
| EPCs | evidence-based practice centers |
| EOD | extent of disease |
| | |
| FACCT | Foundation for Accountability |
| FACT-B | Functional Assessment of Cancer Therapy-Breast quality-of-life instrument |
| FDA | Food and Drug Administration |
| FOIA | Freedom of Information Act of 1966 |
| | |
| HCFA | Health Care Financing Administration |
| HCUP | Healthcare Cost and Utilization Project |
| HEDIS® | Health Plan Employer Data and Information Set |
| HIPAA | Health Insurance Portability and Accountability Act |
| HMO | Health Maintenance Organization |
| | |
| IACR | International Association of Cancer Registries |
| IARC | International Agency for Research on Cancer |
| IHA | Independent Health Association |
| IMSystem® | Indicator Measurement System |
| IOM | Institute of Medicine |
| | |
| JCAHO | Joint Commission on the Accreditation of Healthcare Organizations |
| | |
| NAACCR | North American Association of Centralized Cancer Registries |
| NAMCS | National Ambulatory Medical Care Survey |
| NCCCS | National Coordinating Council for Cancer Surveillance |
| NCCN | National Comprehensive Cancer Network |
| NCDB | National Cancer Data Base |
| NCHS | National Center for Heath Statistics |
| NCI | National Cancer Institute |
| NCQA | National Committee for Quality Assurance |
| NIH | National Institutes of Health |
| NMFS | National Mortality Followback Survey |
| NPCR | National Program of Cancer Registries |
| | |
| PCE | Patient Care Evaluation study |
| PCS | Patterns of Care Study |
| PGBH | Pacific Business Group on Health |
| PPMC | Physician Practice Management Company |
| PPO | preferred provider organization |
| PROs | peer review organizations |
| | |
| QCCC | Quality of Cancer Care Committee |
| QuIC | Quality Interagency Coordination Task Force |

| | |
|---|---|
| Q-Span | expanding and improving quality of care measures |
| SEER | Surveillance, Epidemiology, and End Results program |
| SS | summary stage |
| TNM | tumor, node, metastasis |
| VA | Department of Veterans Affairs |

# APPENDIX A

# *Ensuring Quality Cancer Care:*
# Report Summary

We all want to believe that when people get cancer—including ourselves and our relatives—they will get health care of the highest quality. Concerns about a growing lack of public confidence in the nation's system of care prompted the National Cancer Policy Board to undertake a comprehensive review of the evidence on the effectiveness of cancer services and delivery systems, the adequacy of quality assurance mechanisms, and barriers that impede access to cancer care. The National Cancer Policy Board (NCPB) was established in March 1997 at the Institute of Medicine (IOM) and National Research Council to address issues that arise in the prevention, control, diagnosis, treatment, and palliation of cancer. The 20-member board includes consumers, health care providers, and investigators in several disciplines. The NCPB report, *Ensuring Quality Cancer Care*, addresses five questions:

1. What is the state of the cancer care "system"?
2. What is quality cancer care and how is it measured?
3. What cancer care quality problems are evident and what steps can be taken to improve care?
4. How can we improve what we know about the quality of cancer care?
5. What steps can be taken to overcome barriers to access to quality cancer care?

---

Reproduced from National Cancer Policy Board, *Ensuring Quality Cancer Care,* Washington, D.C.: National Academy Press, 1999.

## WHAT IS THE STATE OF THE CANCER CARE "SYSTEM"?

The National Cancer Policy Board began its deliberations on quality by trying to describe what an ideal cancer care system would look and feel like from the vantage point of an individual receiving cancer care. The NCPB suggested that, for many, excellence in cancer care would be achieved if individuals had:

- access to comprehensive and coordinated services;
- confidence in the experience and training of their providers;
- a feeling that providers respected them, listened to them, and advocated on their behalf;
- an ability to ask questions and voice opinions comfortably, to be full participants in all decisions regarding care;
- a clear understanding of their diagnosis and access to information to aid this understanding;
- awareness of all treatment options and of the risks and benefits associated with each;
- confidence that recommended treatments are appropriate, offering the best chance of a good outcome consistent with personal preferences;
- a prospective plan for treatment and palliation;
- a health care professional responsible (and accountable) for organizing this plan in partnership with each individual; and
- assurances that agreed-upon national standards of quality care are met at their site of care.

The NCPB then described at least some aspects of a cancer care *system* that would support such an ideal state of care. A system of ideal cancer care would

- articulate goals consistent with this vision of quality cancer care;
- implement policies to achieve these goals;
- identify barriers to the practice and receipt of quality care and target interventions to overcome these barriers;
- further efforts to coordinate the currently diverse systems of care;
- ensure appropriate training for cancer care providers;
- have mechanisms in place to facilitate the translation of research to clinical practice;
- monitor and ensure the quality of care; and
- conduct research necessary to further the understanding of effective cancer care.

**The NCPB has concluded that for many Americans with cancer, there is a wide gulf between what could be construed as the ideal and the reality of their experience with cancer care.**

There is no national cancer care program or system of care in the United States. Like other chronic illnesses, efforts to diagnose and treat cancer are centered on individual physicians, health plans, and cancer care centers. The ad hoc and fragmented cancer care system does not ensure access to care, lacks coordination, and is inefficient in its use of resources. The authority to organize, coordinate, and improve cancer care services rests largely with service providers and insurers. At numerous sites in the federal government, programs and research directly relate to the quality of cancer care, but in no one place are these disparate efforts coordinated or even described. Efforts to improve cancer care in many cases will therefore be local or regional and could feasibly originate in a physician's practice, a hospital, or a managed care plan. Because cancer disproportionately affects the elderly, the Medicare program could be an important vehicle for change. Certainly, issues related to quality cancer care have to be addressed at the national and state levels, in coordination with other quality-of-care efforts.

## WHAT IS QUALITY CANCER CARE AND HOW IS IT MEASURED?

Health care can be judged as good to the extent that it increases the likelihood of desired health outcomes and is consistent with current professional knowledge (IOM, 1990). In practical terms, poor quality can mean

- overuse (e.g., unnecessary tests, medication, and procedures, with associated risks and side effects);
- underuse (e.g., not receiving a lifesaving surgical procedure); or
- misuse (e.g., medicines that should not be given together, poor surgical technique).

Quality care means providing patients with appropriate services in a technically competent manner, with good communication, shared decision making, and cultural sensitivity.

The first step in assessing quality of care is establishing which attributes of care are linked to optimal outcomes (e.g., survival, enhanced quality of life). Large, carefully designed clinical trials are usually necessary to establish which specific processes of care or treatments are effective. Early detection of breast cancer through screening mammography, for example, has been shown to reduce mortality significantly for women age 50 and older. Other types of research, notably health services research, also have a role to play in defining high-quality care. Next, observations of current medical practice—for example, through reviews of a sample of medical records—reveal the extent to which effective care is being applied. Measures of quality may assess structural aspects of the health care delivery system (e.g., hospital case volume), processes of care (e.g., use of screening), or outcomes of care (e.g., survival, quality of life). Each of these dimensions of quality could be assessed to provide complementary information.

## WHAT PROBLEMS ARE EVIDENT IN THE QUALITY OF CANCER CARE AND WHAT STEPS CAN BE TAKEN TO IMPROVE CARE?

More is known about the quality of care for breast cancer than for any other kind of cancer. Treatment of early breast cancer saves lives, and early detection through screening contributes to early diagnosis, when treatment is most effective. When established quality measures have been used to assess the care women receive, the following quality problems have been identified:

- underuse of mammography to detect cancer early;
- lack of adherence to standards for diagnosis (e.g., inadequate biopsies, poor reporting of pathology studies);
- inadequate patient counseling regarding treatment options; and
- underuse of radiation therapy and adjuvant chemotherapy after surgery.

The consequences of these lapses in care are, in some cases, reduced survival and, in others, compromised quality of life.

**Based on the best available evidence, some individuals with cancer do not receive care known to be effective for their condition. The magnitude of the problem is not known, but the National Cancer Policy Board believes it is substantial. The reasons for failure to deliver high-quality care have not been studied adequately, nor has there been much investigation of how appropriate standards vary from patient to patient.**

The means for improving the quality of cancer care, which involve changes in the health care system, are the first five of a total of ten recommendations of the National Cancer Policy Board. Implementation of these recommendations may vary by locality and by system of care with, for example, different mechanisms needed in rural versus urban areas, or for particularly high-risk or underserved populations.

Cancer care is optimally delivered in systems of care that:

**RECOMMENDATION 1: Ensure that patients undergoing procedures that are technically difficult to perform and have been associated with higher mortality in lower-volume settings receive care at facilities with extensive experience (i.e., high-volume facilities). Examples of such procedures include removal of all or part of the esophagus, surgery for pancreatic cancer, removal of pelvic organs, and complex chemotherapy regimens.**

Many aspects of the delivery of health care can potentially affect its quality. There is convincing evidence of a relationship between treatment in higher-volume hospitals and better short-term survival for individuals with several types of cancer for which high-risk surgery is indicated (e.g., pancreatic cancer, non-small-cell lung cancer). Several studies show very large effects, with lower-volume hospitals having postsurgical mortality rates two to three times higher than hospitals that do more such procedures. A dose–response effect is also evident to support the finding that as volume increases, so do good outcomes. The findings cut across cancer types and systems of care, sharing the common element of complicated medical or surgical intervention. Although estimates are imprecise, a relatively large share of high-risk surgery is taking place in lower-volume settings (e.g., from one-quarter to one-half of surgical procedures for pancreatic cancer).

More limited data show a relationship between surgery performed at higher-volume hospitals and better outcomes for men with prostate cancer who undergo radical prostatectomy and for women who undergo breast cancer surgery. A few studies of the management of other types of cancer (i.e., testicular cancer, leukemia) also show a relationship between higher volume and better outcome. This volume–outcome relationship appears to be strong, and consistent with findings from other areas of complex care (e.g., coronary revascularization procedures).

**Even in the absence of extensive data for each particular cancer type and stage, evidence strongly indicates that health outcomes are better in high-volume settings for highly technical cancer management.**

**RECOMMENDATION 2: Use systematically developed guidelines based on the best available evidence for prevention, diagnosis, treatment, and palliative care.**

Total quality improvement initiatives, disease management programs, and implementation of clinical practice guidelines all have the potential to improve care within health systems. Information about clinical practice can serve as a powerful tool to change physician and patient behavior and to improve the use of effective treatments. The experience with oncology practice guidelines has been mixed, however, with some examples of success, but other examples of failure to change provider behavior or outcomes. Many guideline efforts have failed because of flaws in the way the guidelines were developed or implemented. Evidence suggests that care can be improved when providers themselves are involved in shaping guidelines and when systems of accountability are in place. Such efforts must be intensified.

**RECOMMENDATION 3: Measure and monitor the quality of care using a core set of quality measures.**

Once effective care has been identified through the research system, mechanisms to develop and implement measurement systems are needed. Translating research results into quality monitoring measures is a complex process that will require significant research investments. There is now a broad consensus about how to assess some aspects of quality of care for many common cancers (e.g., cancers of the breast, colon, lung, prostate, and cervix), but specific measures of the quality of care for these cancers are still being developed and tested within health delivery systems.

Systematic improvements in health care quality will likely only occur through collaborative efforts of the public and private sectors. As large health care purchasers, both sectors have a stake in improving the quality of care, and both sectors have knowledge and experience concerning quality measurement and reporting. A public–private collaborative approach has recently been recommended by the President's Advisory Commission on Consumer Protection and Quality in the Health Care Industry, and some initial implementation steps are being taken (President's Advisory Commission, 1998).

**Cancer care quality measures should span the continuum of cancer care and be developed through a coordinated public–private effort.**

To ensure the rapid translation of research into practice, a mechanism is needed to quickly identify the results of research with quality-of-care implications and ensure that it is applied in monitoring quality. In a few areas, evidence suggests that care does not meet national standards for interventions known to improve care. After primary prevention, cancer screening is the most effective method to reduce the burden of cancer, yet screening is underused. It is often health care providers who can be held accountable for the underuse of cancer screening tests. One of the strongest predictors of whether a person will be screened for cancer is whether the physician recommends it, and evidence suggests that physicians order fewer cancer screening tests than they should. Even when screening is accomplished, many individuals fail to receive timely, or any, follow-up of an abnormal screening test. Both screening and follow-up rates can be improved with interventions aimed both at those eligible for screening and at health care providers (e.g., reminder systems). Implementation of accountability systems can greatly increase participation in cancer screening.

**Cancer care quality measures should be used to hold providers, including health care systems, health plans, and physicians, accountable for demonstrating that they provide and improve quality of care.**

There are many opportunities to exert leverage on the health care system to improve quality. Quality assurance systems are often not apparent to consumers, but have the potential to greatly affect their care:

- large employer groups are holding managed care plans accountable for quality performance goals;
- the Health Care Financing Administration (HCFA, which funds Medicare and the federal component of Medicaid) requires Medicare and Medicaid health plans to produce standard quality reports; and
- state Medicaid programs are beginning to include quality provisions in their contracts with plans and providers.

Six of ten new cancer cases occur among people age 65 and older and, consequently, Medicare is the principal payer for cancer care. There is generally a lack of quality-related data from fee-for-service providers from whom most Medicare beneficiaries receive their care. Information systems are, however, in place that allow the reporting on a regional basis of some quality indicators (e.g., cancer screening rates) relevant to those in fee-for-service systems. For Medicare beneficiaries in managed care plans, accountability systems should incorporate core measures of quality cancer care.

**Cancer care quality measures should be applied to care provided through the Medicare and Medicaid programs as a requirement for participation in these programs.**

The collection, reporting, and analysis of information about the quality of cancer care will be expensive. Many segments of the health care industry will invest in information systems to maximize efficiency and to stay competitive, however, some may require incentives to provide patient-level data.

Information about quality cancer care is becoming more available to individuals with cancer (or at risk for cancer), but it is not yet easily accessible or understandable to consumers. A number of potential quality indicators can be listed, but most have not been evaluated to assess their ultimate value for consumers. It is unclear, for example, how the following indicators affect an individual's experience of care or health care outcomes:

- a physician's board certification,
- a hospital's approval status, for example, as determined by the American College of Surgeons' Commission on Cancer, and
- a health plan's accreditation status and quality scores from the National Committee for Quality Assurance.

By the time a diagnosis of cancer is made and individuals have a clear reason to seek quality care, it is often too late to switch health plans. Also, even if they wanted to, most people do not have access to alternative plans. Individuals may use available quality indicators to choose doctors and hospitals within their plans, and perhaps to choose alternative courses of treatment, but evidence suggests that individual consumers can exert only a modest "market" pressure for quality improvement through access to better information about the quality of cancer care. Large purchasers, such as employers, are likely to exert more leverage and to have designated staff to assess alternative plans.

**Cancer care quality measures should be disseminated widely and communicated to purchasers, providers, consumer organizations, individuals with cancer, policy makers, and health services researchers, in a form that is relevant and useful for health care decision-making.**

Quality measures enable consumers and purchasers to judge the quality of a system of care by its performance relative to evidence-based standards.

**RECOMMENDATION 4: Ensure the following elements of quality care for each individual with cancer:**

- **that recommendations about initial cancer management, which are critical in determining long-term outcome, are made by experienced professionals;**
- **an agreed-upon care plan that outlines goals of care;**
- **access to the full complement of resources necessary to implement the care plan;**
- **access to high-quality clinical trials;**
- **policies to ensure full disclosure of information about appropriate treatment options;**
- **a mechanism to coordinate services; and**
- **psychosocial support services and compassionate care.**

Some elements of care simply make sense—that is, they have strong face validity and can reasonably be assumed to improve care unless and until evidence accumulates to the contrary. This recommendation amounts to a statement of the ideal, based on principles of cancer care articulated by cancer survivors. Details of how to interpret and apply the principles will vary according to health plan, cancer type, stage of disease, and preferences of the individual needing care.

**RECOMMENDATION 5: Ensure quality of care at the end of life, in particular, the management of cancer-related pain and timely referral to palliative and hospice care.**

Cancer is the second leading cause of death in the United States. A strong body of evidence suggests that the experience of dying for many with cancer can be greatly improved with better palliative care (IOM, 1997). Many individuals with cancer suffer pain needlessly and have their treatment preferences ignored. Practice guidelines are available to assist health care providers in this area, but they have not been adopted widely. Financial barriers limit effective care for people at the end of life. Additional studies are needed to identify nonfinancial barriers to appropriate end-of-life care.

## HOW CAN WE IMPROVE WHAT WE KNOW ABOUT THE QUALITY OF CANCER CARE?

For many aspects of cancer care, it is not yet possible to assess quality because the first step in quality assessment has not been taken—the conduct of clinical trials. Consequently, for many types of cancer, answers to the following basic questions are not yet available:

• How frequently should patients be evaluated following their primary cancer therapy, what tests should be included in the follow-up regimen, and who should provide follow-up care?
• What is the most effective way to manage recurrent cancers, or cancers first identified at late stages?

**RECOMMENDATION 6: Federal and private research sponsors such as the National Cancer Institute, the Agency for Health Care Policy and Research, and various health plans should invest in clinical trials to address questions about cancer care management.**

For some questions regarding cancer management, a health services research component could possibly be integrated into a clinical trial designed to assess the efficacy of a new treatment. For other questions, innovative units of randomization could be used, for example, randomizing providers (instead of patients) to test different clinical management strategies. Such trials have been used to assess educational and service delivery topics (e.g., colorectal screening performed by nurse clinicians, counseling patients to quit smoking).

**RECOMMENDATION 7: A cancer data system is needed that can provide quality benchmarks for use by systems of care (such as hospitals, provider groups, and managed care systems).**

Toward that end, in 1999, the National Cancer Policy Board will hold workshops to:

- identify how best to meet the data needs for cancer in light of quality monitoring goals;
- identify financial and other resources needed to improve the cancer data system to achieve quality-related goals; and
- develop strategies to improve data available on the quality of cancer care.

The second step of quality assessment involves surveillance—making sure that evidence regarding what works is applied in practice. Ideally, quality assessment studies would include recently diagnosed individuals with cancer in care settings representative of contemporary practice across the country, using information sources with sufficient detail to allow appropriate comparisons. The available evidence on the quality of cancer care is far from this ideal.

Two national databases are available with which to assess the quality of cancer care, but each has limitations.

1. The Surveillance, Epidemiology, and End Results (SEER) cancer registry, maintained by the National Cancer Institute (NCI), when linked to Medicare and other insurance administrative files, has been valuable in assessing the quality of care for the elderly and other insured populations. It is also useful in identifying a sample of cases for in-depth studies of quality-related issues. The SEER registry, however, covers only 14 percent of the U.S. population in certain geographic locations, so it may not adequately represent the diversity of systems of care. Finding ways to capture measures of process of care, treatment information, and intermediate outcomes—and to improving the timeliness of reporting—would enhance the registry's use in quality assessment.

2. The National Cancer Data Base (NCDB), a joint project of the American College of Surgeons' Commission on Cancer and the American Cancer Society, now holds information on more than half of all newly diagnosed cases of cancer nationwide and includes many of the demographic, clinical, and health system data elements necessary to assess quality of care. A limitation of the NCDB is the absence of complete information on outpatient care. The NCDB has not yet been widely used to assess quality of care, but it has great potential for doing so.

Existing data systems must be enhanced so that questions about quality of care can be answered comprehensively, on a national scale, without delays of many years between data collection and analysis. An effective system would capture information about:

- individuals with cancer (e.g., age, race and ethnicity, socioeconomic status, insurance or health plan coverage);
- their condition (e.g., stage, grade, histological pattern, comorbid conditions);
- their treatment, including significant outpatient treatments (e.g., adjuvant therapy, radiation therapy);
- their providers (e.g., specialty training);
- site of care delivery (e.g., community hospital, cancer center);
- type of care delivery system (e.g., managed care, fee for service); and
- outcomes (e.g., satisfaction, relapse, complications, quality of life, survival time, death).

It may be costly and difficult to obtain all of the desired data elements for all individuals with available sources, so sampling techniques could be used to make the task manageable for targeted studies. Alternatively, it may be feasible to link some databases (e.g., those describing structural aspects of care such as hospital characteristics) to other existing databases. It is unlikely that one single database can meet all of the various objectives of such systems, for example, cancer surveillance, research, and quality monitoring. Data systems need to be monitored to assure accuracy, and should be automated to improve the timeliness of quality data. Data gathered into national databases, in particular, should be made available quickly for analysis by investigators and evaluators.

**RECOMMENDATION 8: Public and private sponsors of cancer care research should support national studies of recently diagnosed individuals with cancer, using information sources with sufficient detail to assess patterns of cancer care and factors associated with the receipt of good care. Research sponsors should also support training for cancer care providers interested in health services research.**

Grants to support the analysis of data that focus on pressing health policy questions, especially about how the organization and financing of cancer care affect the processes and outcomes of care, should be a high priority. Methodologic research is also needed to improve the quality of cancer-related health services research, for example, to develop tools for "case-mix" adjustments to reduce the potential for bias inherent in observational cancer research.

An annual report that provides a description of the status of cancer-related quality-of-care research, and summarizes relevant published literature in the area would serve as a valuable resource for health services researchers and those involved in quality assessment. Such a report would also help organizations set priorities for research, ensure that their research portfolios address important quality-of-care questions, and ensure that their research programs are complementary and coordinated.

## WHAT STEPS CAN BE TAKEN TO OVERCOME BARRIERS OF ACCESS TO QUALITY CANCER CARE?

**RECOMMENDATION 9: Services for the un- and underinsured should be enhanced to ensure entry to, and equitable treatment within, the cancer care system.**

Cancer is among the most expensive conditions to treat, and individuals with cancer and their families invariably bear some of the financial burden. Most individuals diagnosed with cancer are elderly and have Medicare coverage, but an estimated 7 percent of individuals facing a new diagnosis of cancer lack any health insurance at all. For these individuals, cancer can be catastrophic to their finances as well as their health. The problem that affects far more individuals, however, is underinsurance—health plans and insurance coverage offer some, but often incomplete, protection against the high costs of cancer care. High deductibles, copayments or coinsurance, and coverage caps can all contribute to high out-of-pocket expenditures. Medicare, for example, was estimated to cover only 83 percent of typical total charges for lung cancer and 65 percent of charges for breast cancer in 1986. Some individuals have additional protection through other insurers (e.g., Medigap policies or Medicaid), but despite this, the financial burden of cancer can be substantial even among those covered by a health plan. Limits on prescription drug coverage, an expensive and widely used benefit (e.g., outpatient pain medications), are a particular problem for many with cancer because the drugs are often expensive. A limited number of free services or financial assistance programs are available to people with cancer, but they do not substitute for adequate insurance coverage for cancer treatment.

**RECOMMENDATION 10: Studies are needed to find out why specific segments of the population (e.g., members of certain racial or ethnic groups, older patients) do not receive appropriate cancer care. These studies should measure provider and individual knowledge, attitudes, and beliefs, as well as other potential barriers to access to care.**

While access problems persist throughout cancer care, overcoming barriers to screening and early detection is a priority because after primary prevention, the greatest improvements in outcomes will be realized by identifying cancers early, when treatments are most effective. Moreover, initial planning is extremely important for many types of cancer, because failure on the first treatment severely limits subsequent treatment options due to the nature of cancer progression. Evidence suggests that much of the disparity in mortality by race could be reduced by improving access to primary care and cancer screening.

A number of public and private programs have enhanced access to care. The Centers for Disease Control and Prevention's National Breast and Cervical Cancer Early Detection Program provides screening for women unable to afford care. A few states have launched special programs to pay for cancer care for the poor and uninsured (e.g., the Maryland program for women with breast cancer). Many pharmaceutical companies have patient assistance programs to help defray the costs of expensive chemotherapy drugs. These programs and services cannot substitute for adequate insurance coverage for cancer treatment, but they can ease the financial burden for those eligible to receive them.

Although having health insurance coverage improves access, it does not guarantee good care. Several factors other than insurance status and cost can prevent people from "getting to the door" of a health care provider. These include fear of a diagnosis of cancer, distrust of health care providers, language, geography, and difficulties in getting through appointment systems. Incomplete understanding of cancer risk or certain beliefs, such as the belief that one is not at risk or that nothing can be done to change one's fate, may also prevent people from seeking care. Once "in the door," other barriers to access may surface when attempting to navigate the system: for example, getting from a primary care provider to a specialist. Within the system, providers may have difficulty communicating with patients or have insufficient staff to coordinate care and provide all the services patients need. The cancer care system is complex, and different barriers may impede access to care at different phases.

Individuals who have low educational attainment or are members of certain racial or ethnic minority groups face higher barriers to receiving cancer care and tend to have less favorable outcomes than other groups.[*] Limited access to primary care and cancer screening contributes to having cancer diagnosed at latter stages when prognosis is worse. Differences in treatment by race have been well documented; however, it appears that the effect may actually be more closely related to social class than to race.

Those of advanced age also appear to be vulnerable in the cancer care system. Older people are less likely than younger people to receive effective cancer treatments, despite evidence that the elderly can tolerate and benefit from them. Some undertreatment is explained by provider attitudes toward treating the eld-

---

[*]Research in this area sponsored by the National Institutes of Health is addressed in the 1999 IOM report, *The Unequal Burden of Cancer: An Assessment of NIH Research and Programs for Ethnic Minorities and the Medically Underserved* (IOM, 1999).

erly, who are perceived as less w`lling or able to tolerate aggressive treatment. Some undertreatment may also be due to patient preferences and unwillingness to experience the side effects of certain treatments.

## REFERENCES

IOM (Institute of Medicine). 1990. *Medicare: A Strategy for Quality Assurance*, KN Lohr, ed. Washington, D.C.: National Academy Press.

IOM. 1997. *Approaching Death: Improving Care at the End of Life*. MJ Field, CK Cassel, eds. Washington, D.C.: National Academy Press.

IOM. 1999. *The Unequal Burden of Cancer: An Assessment of NIH Research and Programs for Ethnic Minorities and the Medically Underserved*. MA Haynes, BD Smedley, eds. Washington, D.C.: National Academy Press.

President's Advisory Commission on Consumer Protection and Quality in the Health Care Industry. 1998. *Quality First: Better Health Care for All Americans*. Washington, D.C.

# Workshop Agenda and Participants

## ENHANCING DATA SYSTEMS TO IMPROVE THE
## QUALITY OF CANCER CARE

The National Academies
Cecil and Ida Green Building, Room 130
2001 Wisconsin Avenue, N.W.
Washington, D.C.

### AGENDA

**Monday, October 4**

8:00 a.m.–8:30 a.m.   Continental Breakfast

8:30 a.m.–8:45 a.m.   Welcome and Introduction
*Joseph Simone*

### SESSION ONE: OVERVIEW

Evidence-based measures are available to assess cancer care quality, but data systems are not yet in place to give practitioners information on their performance relative to national or regional norms. This presentation will review well-established quality measures, the need for population-based data and monitoring systems, and outstanding health services research questions that remain to be answered with quality-related data.

8:45 a.m.–9:15 a.m.   What Do We Want? Tools for Quality Monitoring
and Health Services Research
*Tom Smith*

### SESSION TWO: USING CANCER REGISTRIES TO
### MONITOR THE QUALITY OF HEALTH CARE

Population-based cancer registries are the foundation of surveillance and cancer control programs. Presentations on how cancer registry data have been and potentially might be applied to quality assessment will be followed by a status report on the Centers for Disease Control and Prevention's National Program of Cancer Registries, the federal effort to bolster the states' cancer surveillance infrastructure. Next, National Cancer Institute staff will describe how the Surveillance, Epidemiology, and End Results (SEER) program has been used to answer important health services research questions. Brief presentations describing of some of the technical, methodological, and legal issues raised in using registry data to monitor healthcare quality will be followed by a discussion that will focus on the merits and limitations of wider applications of quality assessment using cancer registries.

9:15 a.m.–10:00 a.m.  Using State Registry Data to Monitor Healthcare Quality

- Registry-Based Quality Assessments: A Review
  *Bruce Hillner*
- The potential for registry-based quality assessments
  *John Ayanian*

10:00 a.m.–10:30 a.m.  The Status of State Registries
*Dan Miller*

10:30 a.m.–11:00 a.m.  Using SEER to Answer Quality-Related Health Services Research Questions
*Joan Warren*
*Arnold Potosky*

11:00 a.m.–11:15 a.m.  *Coffee Break*

11:15 a.m.–12:30 p.m.  Issues Related to Using Registry Data to Monitor Quality of Care

- The Intersection of Cancer Surveillance and Quality Assessment
  *Linda Harlan*
  *Joseph Lipscomb*
- Data Elements Needed for Quality Assessment
  *Jay Piccirillo*
- Privacy Issues
  *James Hodge*

12:30 p.m.–1:30 p.m.  *Lunch Break*

1:30 p.m.–2:30 p.m.  Discussion: How Can Registry Data be Used to Monitor Quality?
*Tom Tucker*

## SESSION THREE: CANCER CARE DATA AND ACCOUNTABILITY

Information about clinical practice can serve as a powerful tool to change physician and patient behavior and to improve the quality of care. Hospital-reported data have been used to assess patterns of care and to monitor compliance to practice guidelines. The National Cancer Data Base (NCDB), maintained by the American College of Surgeons and American Cancer Society holds promise for assessing progress toward quality improvement because it includes information on the care experience of nearly 60 percent of individuals diagnosed with cancer. The National Comprehensive Cancer Network (NCCN) is an effort on the part of large cancer centers to collect quality data and incorporate them into an ongoing quality improvement program. Presenters will review the status of these quality initiatives and discuss resources needed to assure complete coverage of individuals, their treatments, and outcomes.

The discussion will focus on the strengths and weakness of these programs, the feasibility of setting national or regional quality benchmarks, and the resources needed to ensure acceptance and quality improvement at the local level.

2:30 p.m.–3:30 p.m.   Using Hospital-Based Data to Monitor Physicians and Hospitals

- The National Cancer Data Base
  *Monica Morrow*
- The National Comprehensive Cancer Network
  *Jane Weeks*

3:30 p.m.–4:00 p.m.   Discussion: Implementing Successful Internal Quality Monitoring
*J. Gale Katterhagen*

4:00 p.m.–4:15 p.m.   *Coffee break*

Six in 10 new cases of cancer occur among the elderly. Consequently, the Health Care Financing Administration (HCFA) in administering the Medicare Program has many opportunities to improve the quality of cancer care. The State-based Peer Review Organizations, for example, have conducted a number of assessments of cancer care quality.

4:15 p.m.–5:00 p.m.   HCFA's Use of Cancer Care Quality Data
*Stephen Jencks*

Various professional organizations are involved in accreditation programs to enhance the quality of care. Individuals involved in three such programs will describe them and their inclusion of cancer care measures.

5:00 p.m.–5:30 p.m.     Accreditation Programs

- Health Plans: National Committee for Quality
  Assurance
  *Roger Winn*
- Physicians: American Medical Association
  *Jeffrey Crane*
- Hospitals: Joint Commission on Accreditation of
  Healthcare Organizations and American College of
  Surgeons' Commission on Cancer
  *Monica Morrow*

**Tuesday, October 5**

8:00 a.m.–8:30 a.m.     Continental Breakfast

8:30 a.m.–9:00 a.m.     Summary of Day One
                        *Vivien Chen*
                        *Tom Smith*

## SESSION FOUR: DATA FOR HEALTH SERVICES
## RESEARCH

9:00 a.m.–10:00 a.m.

The National Center for Health Statistics, the Agency for Health Care Policy and Research, and the American Cancer Society are among the sponsors of
large population-based surveys, providing a wealth of opportunities for health
service researchers. Presenters will provide brief overviews of research using
these resources and will discuss their strengths and weaknesses for cancer research. Next, the purpose, scope, and methods of two large cancer survivorship
surveys being launched by the American Cancer Society will be described.
Lastly, we will hear about NCI's HMO Cancer Research Network, an effort to
facilitate collaborative research among managed care organizations. The discussion will focus on resource needs for health services research.

- National Center for Health Statistics, National
  Hospital Discharge Survey
  *Phyllis Wingo*
- Agency for Health Care Policy and Research,
  Healthcare Cost and Utilization Project
  *David Morris*
- American Cancer Society, Cancer Survivorship Surveys
  *Frank Baker*

- National Cancer Institute, HMO Cancer Research Network
  *Martin Brown*

10:00 a.m.–10:30 a.m.  Discussion: Resource Needs for Health Services Research
*Tom Smith*

## SESSION FIVE: CANCER CARE DATA NEEDS

10:30 a.m.–12:30 p.m.  Discussion with NCPB
*Joseph Simone*

- How can we better use what we already have?
- How can we improve available systems to expand quality monitoring efforts and improve the timeliness of analyses?
- What new data initiatives are needed (e.g., linkages, special studies, new collection systems)?
- What organizational, technical, and financial resources are needed?

## PARTICIPANTS

**John Ayanian, M.D., M.P.P.**
Assistant Professor
Harvard Medical School
Departments of Medicine and
    Health Care Policy

**Frank Baker, Ph.D.**
Vice President for Behavioral
    Research
American Cancer Society

**Rachel Ballard-Barbash, M.D., M.P.H.**
Chief, Applied Research Program
Division of Cancer Control and
    Population Sciences
National Cancer Institute

**Martin Brown, Ph.D.**
Chief, Health Services and
    Economics Branch
Applied Research Program
Division of Cancer Control and
    Population Sciences
National Cancer Institute

**Jeffrey Crane, M.D.**
Staff physician
Raleigh Hematology Oncology
    Clinic

**Linda Harlan, Ph.D.**
Epidemiologist
Applied Research Program
Division of Cancer Control and
    Population Sciences
National Cancer Institute

**Bruce Hillner, M.D.**
Professor of Medicine
Medical College of Virginia
Virginia Commonwealth
    University

**James G. Hodge, Jr., J.D., LL.M.**
Greenwall Fellow
Georgetown University Law Center

**Stephen F. Jencks, M.D., M.P.H.**
Senior Clinical Advisor
Health Standards and Quality
    Bureau
Health Care Financing
    Administration

**J. Gale Katterhagen, M.D.**
Medical Director for the Cancer
    Program and Breast Center
Mills-Peninsula Health Services
Medical Director for Quality
Sutter Health

**Joe Lipscomb, Ph.D.**
Chief, Outcomes Research Branch
Applied Research Program
Division of Cancer Control and
    Population Sciences
National Cancer Institute

**Daniel Miller, M.D., M.P.H.**
Chief, Cancer Surveillance Branch
National Center for Chronic
    Disease Prevention and Health
    Promotion
Division of Cancer Prevention and
    Control
Centers for Disease Control and
    Prevention

**David Morris, M.D.**
Clinical Instructor
Department of Radiation Oncology
University of North Carolina

**Monica Morrow, M.D.**
Professor of Surgery
Northwestern University Medical
    School

**Jay F. Piccirillo, M.D.,F.A.C.S.**
Associate Professor and Director
Clinical Outcomes Research Office
Department of Otolaryngology-
    Head and Neck Surgery
Washington University School of
    Medicine

**Arnold Potosky, Ph.D.**
Operations Research Analyst
Health Services and Economics
    Branch Applied Research
    Program
Division of Cancer Control and
    Population Sciences
National Cancer Institute

**Tom Smith, M.D., F.A.C.P.**
Associate Professor of Medicine
    and Health Administration
Medical College of Virginia
Virginia Commonwealth
    University

**Tom Tucker, M.P.H.**
Associate Professor
Department of Health Services
College of Allied Health
    Professions and Department of
    Preventive Medicine and
    Environmental Health
College of Medicine
University of Kentucky

**Jane Weeks, M.D., M.Sc.**
Associate Professor of Medicine
Harvard Medical School
Associate Professor
Health Policy and Management
Harvard School of Public Health

**Joan Warren, Ph.D.**
Epidemiologist
Health Services and Economics
    Branch
Applied Research Program
Division of Cancer Control and
    Population Sciences
National Cancer Institute

**Phyllis Wingo, Ph.D., M.S.**
Director of Surveillance
Department of Epidemiology and
    Surveillance
American Cancer Society

**Roger Winn M.D.**
Chief, Section of Community
    Oncology
Department of Internal Medical
    Specialties
Division of Medicine
U.T. M.D. Anderson Cancer Center

# Summary of Selected Registry-Based Quality Studies

**TABLE C-1** Examples of Cancer Care Quality Studies Using State Cancer Registry Data (published in the last 10 years)

| Author | State/Topic | Design | Conclusion | Comments |
|---|---|---|---|---|
| Wanebo HJ, Cole B, Chung M, et al. Is Surgical Management Compromised in Elderly Patients with Breast Cancer? *Annals of Surgery* 225(5):579–589, 1997. | Rhode Island Patterns of care associated with age among women treated surgically for breast cancer | Screening and treatment patterns assessed for 5,962 women diagnosed with breast cancer between 1987 and 1995 identified through the state registry (study limited to the 9 institutions using AJCC tumor classification). Descriptive statistics for treatment by age and stage (no comorbidity measures). | Breast cancer management is compromised in the elderly. Detection rate of preinvasive cancers in women 65+ was 8.8% vs. 13.7% for women 40–65. Lumpectomy alone was done in 25.0% of elderly patients with stage I cancer vs. 9.5% in patients 40–65. Lumpectomy alone was done in 9.5% of stage II and 10.6% of stage III in patients 65+ vs. 2.7% and 2.2%, respectively, in younger patients. | The study was not population-based and was limited to those institutions with AJCC tumor classification. No data on comorbidity available. |
| Adams-Cameron M, Gilliland FD, Hunt WC, et al. Trends in Incidence and Treatment for Ductal Carcinoma in Situ in Hispanic, American Indian, and Non-Hispanic White Women in New Mexico, 1973–1994. *Cancer* 85(5):1084–1090, 1999. | New Mexico Patterns of care associated with race/ethnicity among women with ductal carcinoma in situ (DCIS) | Treatment patterns assessed for 950 cases of DCIS identified through the state cancer registry from 1973 to 1994. Patient characteristics included: age at diagnosis, ethnicity, residence, and poverty status (as determined by census tract of residence). Physician characteristics included: age, gender, specialty, volume of surgical breast carcinoma patients, and location of treatment. | The use of BCS for DCIS increased to 52% by 1994. Geographic location of treatment was the most significant predictor of treatment. Other patient and provider characteristics were not related to use of breast-conserving surgery (BCS). | The variation in rates of BCS by treatment location most likely reflects differences in physician practices and treatment recommendations. |

| Hand R, Sener S, Imperato J, et al. Hospital Variables Associated with Quality of Care for Breast Cancer Patients. *JAMA* 226(24):3429–3432, 1991. | Illinois Hospital characteristics potentially affecting compliance with clinical standards for care of breast cancer | Analysis of cancer registry data on 5,766 patients diagnosed in 1988, treated at 99 Illinois hospitals. Five quality indicators studied: proportion of patients diagnosed at late stage, hormone receptor determination, adjuvant therapy, radiation therapy, and axillary lymph node dissection. | Urban location, small size, and marginal reimbursement were related to late diagnosis and inadequate treatment of breast cancer at some hospitals. Nonsignificant hospital variables were proportion of oncology cases and teaching status of hospital. | Few teaching hospitals were included. The study did not address individual patient or physician factors, or lack of payment by insurance. Concurrence on efficiency of treatments and delayed incorporation of new findings into standard care may have influenced hospital practices. Some hospital factors, such as size, setting, and reimbursement, may limit the resources available for cancer care. |
| Desch CE, Penberthy L, Newschaffer CJ, et al. Factors that Determine the Treatment for Local and Regional Prostate Cancer. *Medical Care* 34 (2):152–162, 1996. | Virginia Significance of comorbid and nonclinical factors in prostate cancer care | Three treatment alternatives evaluated for 3,117 men diagnosed between 1985 and 1989: treatment vs. no treatment, surgery vs. radiation, hormonal/orchiectomy vs. surgery/radiation. In addition to comorbidity, other nonclinical factors studied were age, race, residence, and socioeconomic status. Data from linkages of state registry to Medicare claim files, the Area Resource File, and 1990 Census Data. | Age was the most important factor in treatment decisions, even after adjustments for comorbidity. Older men received less treatment as compared with any treatment, less surgery than radiation, and more hormonal therapy than surgery and/or radiation. Other nonclinical factors did impact treatment choices, but to a lesser degree. | Limitations of the data include imprecise staging variables, lack of data on Virginia residents treated in bordering states, and lack of information on physician attributes or patient preferences. |

*Continued*

**TABLE C-1** *Continued*

| Author | State/Topic | Design | Conclusion | Comments |
|---|---|---|---|---|
| Polednak AP. Predictors of Breast-Conserving Surgery in Connecticut, 1990–1992. *Annals of Surgical Oncology* 4(3):259–263, 1997. | Connecticut Sociodemographic characteristics associated with use of BCS | Analysis of predictors of BCS use (poverty status, age at diagnosis, race, marital status, extent of disease, year of diagnosis, and town of residence) among 5,266 women diagnosed in 1990–1992 with early-stage breast cancer. Data from state registry and census tract. | BCS was not associated with poverty level of area of residence, but was lower for larger or node-positive cancers. | Attitudes and practices of local physicians were hypothesized as being important in explaining variation in BCS use by town of residence. High BCS rates (69–94% vs. 49% statewide) were found for residents of a cluster of seven contiguous towns associated with a single hospital. |
| Polednak AP, Shevchenko IP, Flannery JT, et al. 1996. Estimating Breast Cancer Treatment Charges in Connecticut. *Connecticut Medicine* 60(5): 263–267, 1996. | Connecticut Treatment costs for breast cancer | Study assessed charges, which generally exceed actual costs or payments. Random sample of 407 breast cancer patients (all ages) diagnosed in 1991 identified in cancer registry and linked to hospital-discharge database through 1993; 93% of cases linked. | Average charges declined with age, increased with extent of disease (stage at diagnosis), and increased with extent of surgery. | The linked database is most useful in estimating charges for cancers treated mainly by surgery (including ambulatory surgery at hospitals) and for charges associated with comorbid conditions and terminal care. Radiotherapy and most chemotherapy are provided on an outpatient basis, and charges were not reflected in the hospital discharge database. |

| | | | |
|---|---|---|---|
| Hillner BE, McDonald MK, Penberthy L, et al. Measuring Standards of Care for Early Breast Cancer in an Insured Population. *Journal of Clinical Oncology* 15(4):1401–1408, 1997. | Virginia Process of care for women with early breast cancer | 918 women with local/regional invasive breast cancer identified through linking the state registry, 1989–1991, and procedural and hospital claims from Blue Cross Blue Shield (BCBS) of Virginia. Standards of care based upon consensus conferences and literature reviews, quality targets established by the authors. | Achievement of objectives or performance standards varied. For women age 50 or younger, 85% with positive axillary nodes had chemotherapy claims. For older women with positive axillary nodes, 53% had chemotherapy claims. 79% of women had a follow-up mammography within the first 18 months postoperatively. | The state registry collected data on a voluntary basis from approximately 50 hospitals representing about 85% of the state's hospital beds. Some limitations of claims data for quality assessment include: lost claims, the potential bundling of services in the hospital claim, and changes in individual's insurance coverage. |
| Smith TJ, Penberthy L, Desch CE, et al. Differences in Initial Treatment Patterns and Outcomes of Lung Cancer in the Elderly. *Lung Cancer* 13:235–252, 1995. | Virginia Patterns of care among elderly persons with lung cancer | Incident cases of non-small-cell lung cancer (NSCLC) from the state cancer registry, 1985–1989, were matched with claims from Medicare Part A and B ($n = 4,999$), census tract data, and the Area Resource File. Multiple logistic regression analyses used to identify factors associated with therapy choices (controlling for comorbidity). | Older age increased the likelihood of exclusion from potentially curative surgery, even after controlling for other factors. | Less than 10% of patients had TNM staging; however, the locoregional-distant classification works well to estimate survival for lung cancer. |

*Continued*

**TABLE C-1** *Continued*

| Author | State/Topic | Design | Conclusion | Comments |
|---|---|---|---|---|
| Hillner B, Penberthy L, Desch CE, et al. Variation in Staging and Treatment of Local and Regional Breast Cancer in the Elderly. *Breast Cancer Research and Treatment* 40:75–86, 1996. | Virginia Patterns of care among elderly women with local and regional breast cancer | State cancer registry data were linked with Medicare claims and 1990 census data. 3,361 women identified with pathologic confirmed local and regional breast cancer in 1985–1989. Processes of care assessed: tumor size determination, axillary lymph node dissection, use of adjuvant therapy, radiation if BCS was performed. Multivariate analyses including comorbidity. | Older women were more likely to present with larger tumors but were less likely to undergo an axillary node dissection, to receive chemotherapy, or to receive radiation therapy if treated with BCS. | The state registry collected data on a voluntary basis from approximately 50 hospitals representing about 85% of the state's hospital beds. Only 55% of cases had complete TNM staging. A summary staging system (local, regional, and distant disease) was used from the registry. |
| Polednak AP and Flannery JT. Black Versus White Racial Differences in Clinical Stage at Diagnosis and Treatment of Prostatic Cancer in Connecticut. *Cancer* 70(8):2152–2158, 1992. | Connecticut Racial differences in patterns of prostate cancer care | First course of treatment examined by clinical stage for black (localized, *n* = 133; metastases, *n* = 102) and white (localized *n* = 2,653; metastases, *n* = 1,083) men diagnosed with prostate cancer from 1985–1988. Data from CT cancer registry. | There is little difference in therapy received by black versus white patients with prostatic cancer at a given stage of diagnosis. | SEER registries limited by inadequate information on clinical stage and comorbidity. This reduces the ability to interpret the appropriateness of treatment (or lack of treatment) in comparison with ad hoc studies using hospital records. |

Katz SJ, Hislop G, Thomas DB, et al. Delay from Symptom to Diagnosis and Treatment of Breast Cancer in Washington State and British Columbia. *Medical Care* 1(3):264–268, 1993.

Washington, British Columbia (BC), Canada
Delay in time between symptom to diagnosis for women with breast cancer

10% random sample of women 35–80 years old diagnosed with invasive nonmetastatic breast cancer in 1988 in western WA (n = 174) and BC (n = 195). Data from population-based registries assessed for: (1) time from first appearance of symptoms (date of physical exam (PE) or mammography for those without symptoms) to first physician contact; (2) time from first contact to definitive diagnosis by either aspiration or biopsy; and (3) time from definitive diagnosis to initial surgery. Information from medical record review.

Median delay times from first symptom to definitive treatment were short and similar in the two regions. 13.4% of women in Washington and 4.6% of women in BC experienced a diagnosis delay of three months or longer. The higher rate in Washington is explained by greater use of screening mammography and a higher frequency of nonsuspicious diagnostic mammograms.

Because this study only included women who were ultimately diagnosed with breast cancer, the results cannot be generalized to all women presenting with breast-related problems. Another limitation to the study is that medical records may not accurately reflect the onset of symptoms. The impact of delay on prognosis remains uncertain, but delays have negative psychological consequences for women during the diagnostic process. Many patients, for example, have anxiety provoked by equivocal mammographic findings. Physicians are at risk for malpractice claims as a result of a delayed diagnosis of breast cancer.

*Continued*

**TABLE C-1** *Continued*

| Author | State/Topic | Design | Conclusion | Comments |
|---|---|---|---|---|
| Howe HL, Katterhagen JG, Yates J, et al. Urban–rural Differences in the Management of Breast Cancer. *Cancer Causes and Control* 3:533–539, 1992. | Illinois<br><br>Urban–rural differences in patterns of breast cancer care | Cancer management described for women diagnosed with breast cancer in 1986–1987, relative to standards described in NCI's Physician Data Query. Cases grouped as follows: 147 rural residents treated in a local hospital, 119 rural residents treated in an urban hospital, and 451 urban residents treated in a local hospital. Cases identified through the state registry, and management data were obtained via hospital record audit and physician survey. Odds ratios for treatment use adjusted for age and stage. | Rural cases diagnosed in rural hospitals were less likely than urban patients to have staged tumors and more likely to have node dissections. Rural cases traveling to urban centers were less likely to have limited surgery, hormone therapy, and a biopsy as a first step surgical procedure, and more likely to have node dissection.<br><br>Differential urban–rural access to state-of-the-art care contributes to the differential urban–rural rates in breast-cancer case fatality. | Referral networks and potential clustering of specific management practices were assessed by individual physician, surgeon, and hospital of diagnosis. Six of the 61 rural physicians saw one third of the rural patients. Their management practices were similar to other rural physicians except for axillary node dissection and hormone therapy. |

*Continued*

| Ayanian JZ, Kohler BA, Abe T, et al. The Relation Between Health Insurance Coverage and Clinical Outcomes among Women with Breast Cancer. *New England Journal of Medicine* 329(5):326–331, 1993. | New Jersey Effect of insurance status on clinical outcomes for women with breast cancer | Stage of disease and stage-specific survival assessed among 4,675 women, 35–64 years of age, diagnosed with invasive breast cancer between 1985 and 1987. Data from linking state registry records to hospital-discharge data. Survival assessed through 1992. | Uninsured patients and those covered by Medicaid presented with more advanced disease than did privately insured patients. Survival was worse for uninsured patients and those with Medicaid coverage than for privately insured patients with local disease and regional disease, but not distant metastases. | Treatment patterns not assessed. |
|---|---|---|---|---|
| Mann BA, Samet JM, Hunt WC et al. Changing Treatment of Breast Cancer in New Mexico From 1969 Through 1985. *JAMA* 259(23):3413–3417, 1988. | New Mexico Temporal changes in patterns of breast cancer care | Treatment within four months of diagnosis was assessed for 6,030 women diagnosed with primary breast cancer (local or regional) from 1969 through 1985 as identified in the state cancer registry. To assure accurate classification of the use of radiotherapy, files of patients recorded as having undergone BCS or simple mastectomy without radiotherapy were reviewed. In addition, records of radiotherapy facilities within the state were reviewed. No information available on comorbidity. | Use of BCS rose from 6% to 25% after 1980. Women younger than 50 or older than 80 were most likely to undergo BCS. Radiotherapy could not be documented for 26% of women 65 years old or younger, or for 56% of the women aged 65 years or older. | The behavior of individual physicians was assessed. During 1981 to 1984, all but 7 of 43 surgeons actively involved in breast cancer surgery had performed at least one BCS. Twenty surgeons used the procedure in >10% of their patient population. The use of BCS did not correlate with the surgeon's age, volume of cases, or use of BCS before 1981. |

**TABLE C-1** *Continued*

| Author | State/Topic | Design | Conclusion | Comments |
|---|---|---|---|---|
| Roohan PJ, Bickell NA, Baptiste MS, et al. Hospital Volume Difference and Five-Year Survival from Breast Cancer. *American Journal of Public Health* 88(3):454–457, 1998. | New York Effect of hospital volume of BCS cases on the 5-year survival of women treated for breast cancer | Assessment of 5-year survival and risk of death for 47,890 women, diagnosed between 1984 and 1989, identified through linkages between the NY hospital discharge database and the state registry. Adjustments made for surgery type, cancer stage, comorbidity, age, race, socioeconomic status, and distance to hospital. Hospital volume classified in four groups, ranging from very low (10 or fewer cases) to high (150 BCS performed per year). | Unadjusted 5-year survival rates were significantly higher at high-volume hospitals, for each cancer stage. Patients at very low-volume hospitals had a 60% higher risk of death than patients at high-volume hospitals. Patients at low- (11–50 cases) and moderate- (51–150) volume hospitals had 30% and 19%, respectively, higher risks of dying. | The "dose-response" relationship between volume and survival supports a causal relationship. Limitations of administrative databases are reflected in limitations of the study. Socioeconomic status was not measured as the individual level. It was based on contextual data—address of residence. Comorbidity measurements may not accurately reflect severity, so adjustment may have been incomplete. |

# APPENDIX D

# Information on
# Cancer Registries, by State

**TABLE D-1** State Cancer Registries—Indicators of Data Quality

| State[a] | General Information | | Data Quality Indicators | | | | Year Casefinding[g] Began Using: | |
|---|---|---|---|---|---|---|---|---|
| | Year of Initial Operation | Year Population-Based Data[b] Available | Death Certificate Only (%)[c] | Estimate of Completeness (%)[d] | Included in U.S. Combined Rates?[e] | Certified in 1999?[f] | M.D. Offices | Ambulatory Surgical Centers |
| Arizona | 1981 | 1995 | 2.2 | 86.0 | | ✓ | 1992 | 1992 |
| California | 1946 | 1988 | 1.2 | 100.4 | ✓ | ✓ | 1988 | 1988 |
| Colorado | 1968 | 1988 | 1.8 | 102.2 | ✓ | ✓ | 1995 | 1988 |
| Connecticut | 1935 | 1935 | 1.5 | 108.9 | ✓ | ✓ | No | No |
| Delaware | 1972 | 1972 | 5.7 | 92.9 | ✓ | | 1998 | No |
| Florida | 1981 | 1981 | NA | 99.7 | ✓ | | No | 1995 |
| Hawaii | 1960 | 1960 | 0.4 | 112.8 | ✓ | ✓ | 1960 | 1978 |
| Idaho | 1969 | 1970 | 1.7 | 101.1 | ✓ | ✓ | 1980 | 1988 |
| Illinois | 1985 | 1986 | 5.4 | 93.0 | ✓ | ✓ | No | 1994 |
| Indiana | 1987 | 1987 | NA | NA | | | No | No |
| Iowa | 1973 | 1973 | 1.2 | 101.9 | ✓ | ✓ | No | 1988 |
| Kentucky | 1991 | 1991 | 3.2 | 90.6 | ✓ | ✓ | No | 1995 |
| Louisiana | 1974 | 1988 | 1.6 | 94.4 | ✓ | ✓ | 1995 | 1988 |
| Maine | 1983 | 1983 | NA | 89.5 | | | 1995 | 1995 |
| Maryland | 1982 | 1982 | NA | NA | | | 1996 | 1996 |
| Massachusetts | 1980 | 1982 | NA | 91.0 | ✓ | | No | 1982 |
| Michigan | 1985 | 1985 | 1.2 | 99.4 | ✓ | | No | No |
| Minnesota | 1988 | 1988 | 1.0 | 98.8 | ✓ | ✓ | No | No |

| | | | | | | | |
|---|---|---|---|---|---|---|---|
| Montana | 1979 | NA | 83.5 | | | No | No |
| Nebraska | 1987 | 0.3 | 92.0 | | ✓ | 1990 | No |
| Nevada | 1979 | 2.0 | NA | | | No | 1990 |
| New Hampshire | 1987 | NA | 89.4 | | | 1986 | 1987 |
| New Jersey | 1979 | 2.7 | 99.0 | ✓ | ✓ | 1978 | 1988 |
| New Mexico | 1973 | 2.0 | 94.9 | ✓ | ✓ | 1973 | 1973 |
| New York | 1976 | 4.8 | 93.3 | | | No | No |
| North Carolina | 1990 | NA | 89.0 | | | 1990 | 1995 |
| Pennsylvania | 1985 | NA | 97.2 | | | No | No |
| Rhode Island | 1986 | 2.1 | 101.3 | ✓ | ✓ | 1986 | 1986 |
| Tennessee | 1989 | NA | NA | | | No | No |
| Texas | 1992 | 6.5 | 92.9 | | | No | No |
| Utah | 1966 | 0.2 | 98.7 | ✓ | ✓ | 1973 | 1994 |
| Virginia | 1970 | NA | 81.5 | | | 1998 | 1998 |
| Washington | 1991 | 3.5 | 103.4 | ✓ | ✓ | 1992 | 1992 |
| West Virginia | 1993 | 2.1 | 92.5 | ✓ | ✓ | No | 1993 |
| Wisconsin | 1978 | 3.7 | 103.8 | ✓ | | 1992 | 1992 |
| Wyoming | 1962 | 0.4 | 91.0 | ✓ | | 1962 | 1997 |

[a]Thirty-six state registries responded to NAACCR's *Call for Data*. The nonparticipating registries include: Alaska, Alabama, Arkansas, Georgia, Kansas, Mississippi, Missouri, North Dakota, Ohio, Oklahoma, Oregon, South Carolina, South Dakota, and Vermont.
[b]A population-based registry is defined as one that "includes information about all cases of a specific disease in a geographically defined area that relates to a specific population." [From: Wallace RB (ed). *Maxcy, Rosenau, Last-Public Health and Preventive Medicine*, 14th ed. Stamford, CT: Appleton and Lange, 1998.]

*Continued*

144

**TABLE D-1** *Continued*

[c]*Standards for Cancer Registries*, Vol. III, p. 41. Based on the experience of the SEER Program, 1%–1.5% death-certificate-only (DCO) cases are expected and acceptable. Values between 0% and 1% or 1.5% and 3% require analysis and explanation. If 0% are DCO, death clearance has not been performed. A high percentage of DCO cases may be the result of underreporting from other sources, incomplete investigation (or follow back) of the DCO cases due to limited resources, or both. In addition, when a population-based registry first begins death clearance, the percentage of DCO cases tends to be higher because some DCO cases were diagnosed prior to the operation of the registry and therefore are not linked to the registry database.

[d]Vol. I: *Incidence*, p. I-7. The adjusted NAACCR estimate of completeness was calculated using the following equation:

$$\text{Adjusted \% Completeness} = (\text{Observed } C_s - D_s) \times 100\%$$

$$\text{Expected } C_s$$

where observed $C_s$ = number of cancer cases for all sites in the registry, $D_s$ = number of duplicate records (calculated using the NAACCR estimate of duplicates, based on the registry's results from completing the *Protocol for Assessing Duplicate Cases*), and Expected $C_s$ = estimated number of cancer for all sites if completeness is 100%. [See Vol. I: *Incidence*, pp. 7–8 for a detailed derivation of this equation and its variables.]

For registries that did not complete the *Protocol for Assessing Duplicate Cases*, the NAACCR adjusted estimate for completeness is omitted from the registry description.

[e]Indicates states which meet all the following criteria for inclusion in the U.S. combined rates (Vol. I: *Incidence*, pp. 6–8):

1. Data for all 5 years, 1991–1995, were submitted.
2. The registry completed the *Protocol for Assessing Duplicate Cases*, developed by the Data Evaluation and Publication Committee, and submitted the results. If a registry had an estimate of duplicates that exceeded one per 1,000 records or 0.1%, given its required sample size, the registry was not eligible for inclusion in the combined rates.

3. The registry ran the case records for 1991–1995 against the *Call for Data* metafile prepared for the EDITS software and made all corrections.

4. The completeness of case ascertainment was completed using the formula above. Every registry included in the combined rates had an adjusted completeness estimate of at least 90%. The computed completeness estimate for all registries included in the combined incidence rates for the United States was about 99%.

*f*See Table D-2 for certification criteria. Registries were certified in 1,000 based on cases reported as of 1996.

*g*This date indicates the first year that cancer cases were reported from various sources. In addition to physicians' offices and ambulatory surgical centers, which are included in this summary table, cancer cases were also reported from the following sources: hospitals, death certificates, nonhospital pathology labs, radiation therapy sites, interstate data exchange, and nursing homes/hospices. Complete data for these sources can be found in the monograph.

SOURCES:
Chen VW, Wu XC, Andrews PA (eds.). 1999. *Cancer in North America: 1991–1995. Volume One: Incidence.* Sacramento, CA: NAACCR.
Tucker TC, HL Howe and HK Weir. 1999. Certification for population-based registries. *J Registry Manage* Feb:24–27.

**TABLE D-2** North American Association of Central Cancer Registries (NAACCR) Criteria and Standards for Certification of Cancer Registries

| Criteria | Measure | Rationale | Gold Standard | Silver Standard |
|---|---|---|---|---|
| Completeness of case ascertainment | 1. Compare actual incidence rate to expected incidence rate, using SEER Incidence to U.S. mortality ratio method* | Demonstrates the registry has identified a sufficient proportion of expected cases. | 95% completeness | 90% completeness |
| | 2. Death clearance: Match all cancer deaths with registry records, and follow back on unmatched cancer deaths | Provides a more accurate count of cancer incidence by looking at unmatched cancer deaths. | Complete death clearance | Complete death clearance |
| | 3. Number of duplicate records | Duplicates should be consolidated to ensure that one case is not entered more than once from different institutions. | <1 duplicate per 1,000 | <2 duplicates per 1,000 |
| Completeness of information recorded | 1. Sociodemographic Information (% missing) | Includes: age at diagnosis, sex, race, county of residence at diagnosis | <2% missing (3% for race) | <3% missing (5% for race) |
| | 2. Percentage of "death certificate only" (DCO) cases | DCO cases often lack information on key variables, which limits utility, so a minimal proportion of DCO cases is desired. | <3% | <5% |

| | | | | |
|---|---|---|---|---|
| Accuracy of data | EDITS metafile: an electronic editing procedure capable of identifying logical inconsistencies in case records | Ensures that information is consistent and accurate enough to be useful. | 99% cases passing EDITS | 97% cases passing EDITS |
| Timeliness | All information and corrections must be entered within 23 months from close of diagnosis year. | Timely submission of information | Data submitted | Data submitted |

NOTE: For certification at either the gold or silver standard, a registry must meet all criteria for that particular level of certification.

*The incidence to mortality ratio method uses the ratio of SEER incidence (site, race, and sex-specific) to U.S. mortality, and applies that ratio to the site, race, and sex-specific mortality rates of the population served by the registry. The expected incidence rate is calculated by multiplying these rate ratios by the cancer-specific mortality rate for that population. The incidence to mortality rate ratio method provides a more accurate expected incidence rate because it allows for the possibility that different populations have lower incidence rates. In the past, expected incidence was calculated by applying incidence rates of one area with complete case ascertainment, to the area under evaluation; this method assumed that the cancer incidence rates were similar.

SOURCE: Tucker TC, HL Howe and HK Weir. Certification for Population-Based Cancer Registries. *J Registry Management.* Feb 1999: 24–27.

APPENDIX E

# Reporting Requirements, NPCR, NCDB, SEER,

SOURCE: Commission on Cancer, 1996. *Standards of the Commission on Cancer, Volume II: Registry Operations and Data Standards.* Chicago: Commission on Cancer. Reprinted with permission.

## DEFINITIONS

**Required Data Set (R)**

Commission-approved programs must record the required data set items using the codes and definitions specified in the ROADS.

**Supplementary Data Set (S)**

The supplementary data set contains additional data items that are important for the efficient operation of a cancer registry. The Commission recommends that the supplementary data set be collected.

**Optional Data Set (O)**

The optional data set includes items that may be of interest to specific institutions or groups.

**Surveillance, Epidemiology, and End Results Program (SEER)**

Required data elements for a central registry affiliated with the National Cancer Institute's SEER Program.

**National Program of Cancer Registries (NPCR)**

Required and recommended data elements for state cancer registries participating in the National Program of Cancer Registries of the Centers for Disease Control & Prevention.

## COMPARISON OF DATA SETS

An (x) indicates that the item is part of the data set.

*At the time of publication, it is unknown if the organization will collect this data item.

| ITEM | COC | | | SEER | NPCR |
|---|---|---|---|---|---|
| | R | S | O | | |
| **PATIENT IDENTIFICATION** | | | | | |
| Institution ID number (Required for participants in multiple-hospital registries) | x | | | | |
| Accession number | x | | | x | x |
| Sequence number | x | | | x | x |
| Year first seen for this primary | x | | | | |
| Medical record number | x | | | | x |
| Social Security number | x | | | | x |
| Military medical record number suffix | | x | | | x |
| Name, prefix | | | x | | |
| Name, suffix | | x | | | |
| Last name | x | | | | x |
| First name | x | | | | x |
| Middle name | x | | | | x |

*Section Three: Comparison of Data Sets*

| ITEM | R | S | O | SEER | NPCR |
|------|---|---|---|------|------|
| Maiden name | | x | | | x |
| Alias | | x | | | x |
| Marital status at diagnosis | | | x | x | x |
| Patient address (number and street) at diagnosis | x | | | | x |
| City/town at diagnosis | x | | | | x |
| State at diagnosis | x | | | | x |
| Postal code at diagnosis | x | | | | x |
| County at diagnosis | x | | | x | x |
| Patient address (number and street) - current | x | | | | |
| City/Town - current | x | | | | |
| State - current | x | | | | |
| Postal code - current | x | | | | |
| County - current | | | x | | |
| Census tract | | | x | x | x |
| Census coding system | | | x | x | x |
| Telephone | x | | | | |
| Place of birth | | | x | x | x |
| Date of birth | x | | | x | x |
| Age at diagnosis | | x | | x | x |
| Race | x | | | x | x |
| Spanish Origin | x | | | x | x |
| Sex | x | | | x | x |
| Following physician | x | | | | |
| Managing physician | | x | | | |
| Primary surgeon | x | | | | |
| Physician #3 | | x | | | |
| Physician #4 | | x | | | |
| Primary payer at diagnosis | x | | | | |
| Usual occupation | | | x | | x |
| Usual industry | | | x | | x |
| Family history of cancer | | | x | | |
| Tobacco history | | | x | | |
| Alcohol history | | | x | | |
| Type of reporting source | | | x | x | x |
| Abstracted by | x | | | | |

*Section Three: Comparison of Data Sets*

| ITEM | COC | | | SEER | NPCR |
|------|-----|---|---|------|------|
| | R | S | O | | |
| **CANCER IDENTIFICATION** | | | | | |
| Class of case | x | | | | x |
| Institution referred from | | x | | | |
| Institution referred to | | x | | | |
| Date of inpatient admission | | x | | | |
| Date of inpatient discharge | | x | | | |
| Inpatient/outpatient status | | | x | | |
| Screening date | | | x | | |
| Screening result | | | x | | |
| Date of initial diagnosis | x | | | x | x |
| Primary site | x | | | x | x |
| Laterality | x | | | x | x |
| Histology | x | | | x | x |
| Behavior code | x | | | x | x |
| Grade/differentiation | x | | | x | x |
| Diagnostic confirmation | x | | | x | x |
| Tumor marker #1 | | x | | x | |
| Tumor marker #2 | | x | | x | |
| Tumor marker #3 | | x | | * | * |
| Presentation at cancer conference | | x | | | |
| Date of cancer conference | | | x | | |
| Referral to support services | | x | | | |
| **STAGE OF DISEASE AT DIAGNOSIS** | | | | | |
| Size of tumor | x | | | x | x |
| Extension (SEER EOD) | | x | | x | |
| Lymph nodes (SEER EOD) | | x | | x | |
| Regional nodes examined | x | | | x | |
| Regional nodes positive | x | | | x | |
| Site of distant metastasis #1 | | x | | | |
| Site of distant metastasis #2 | | x | | | |
| Site of distant metastasis #3 | | x | | | |
| General Summary Stage (SEER) (Required only in the absence of AJCC classification) | x | | | | x |
| Clinical T | x | | | | |
| Clinical N | x | | | | |
| Clinical M | x | | | | |
| Clinical stage group | x | | | | |
| Clinical stage (prefix/suffix) descriptor | | x | | | |
| Staged by (clinical stage) | x | | | | |
| Pathologic T | x | | | | |

*Section Three: Comparison of Data Sets*

| ITEM | COC | | | SEER | NPCR |
|---|---|---|---|---|---|
| | R | S | O | | |
| Pathologic N | x | | | | |
| Pathologic M | x | | | | |
| Pathologic stage group | x | | | | |
| Pathologic stage (prefix/suffix) descriptor | | x | | | |
| Staged by (pathologic stage) | x | | | | |
| Other T | | x | | | |
| Other N | | x | | | |
| Other M | | x | | | |
| Other stage group | | x | | | |
| Other stage (prefix/suffix) descriptor | | x | | | |
| Staged by (other stage) | x | | | | |
| Other staging system | | | x | | |
| Type of staging system (pediatric) | x | | | | |
| Pediatric stage | x | | | | |
| Staged by (pediatric stage) | x | | | | |
| TNM edition number | x | | | | |
| Date of first positive biopsy | | | x | | |
| Diagnostic and staging procedures | x | | | | |
| **FIRST COURSE OF TREATMENT** | | | | | |
| Date of first course treatment | x | | | x | x |
| Date of non cancer-directed surgery | x | | | | |
| Non cancer-directed surgery | x | | | | |
| Non cancer-directed surgery at this facility | | x | | | |
| Date of cancer-directed surgery | x | | | | x |
| Surgical approach | x | | | * | * |
| Surgery of primary site | x | | | * | * |
| Cancer-directed surgery at this facility | | x | | * | * |
| Surgical margins | x | | | * | * |
| Scope of regional lymph node surgery | x | | | * | * |
| Number of regional lymph nodes removed | x | | | * | * |
| Surgery of other regional site(s), distant site(s) or distant lymph node(s) | x | | | * | * |
| Reconstruction/restoration-first course | x | | | * | * |
| Reason for no surgery | | x | | x | x |
| Date radiation started | x | | | | x |
| Radiation | x | | | x | x |
| Radiation at this facility | | x | | | |
| Regional dose: cGy | | | x | | |
| Number of treatments to this volume | | | x | | |
| Radiation elapsed treatment time (days) | | | x | | |

Section Three: Comparison of Data Sets

| ITEM | COC | | | SEER | NPCR |
|---|---|---|---|---|---|
| | R | S | O | | |
| Radiation treatment volume | | | x | | |
| Location of radiation treatment | | | x | | |
| Intent of treatment (radiation) | | | x | | |
| Regional treatment modality | | | x | | |
| Radiation therapy to CNS | | | x | x | x |
| Radiation/surgery sequence | | | x | x | x |
| Radiation treatment completion status | | | x | | |
| Radiation therapy local control status | | | x | | |
| Reason for no radiation | | x | | | |
| Date chemotherapy started | x | | | | x |
| Chemotherapy | x | | | x | x |
| Chemotherapy at this facility | | x | | | |
| Chemotherapy field #1 | | x | | | |
| Chemotherapy field #2 | | x | | | |
| Chemotherapy field #3 | | x | | | |
| Chemotherapy field #4 | | x | | | |
| Reason for no chemotherapy | | x | | | |
| Date hormone therapy started | x | | | | x |
| Hormone therapy | x | | | x | x |
| Hormone therapy at this facility | | x | | | |
| Reason for no hormone therapy | | x | | | |
| Date immunotherapy started | x | | | | x |
| Immunotherapy | x | | | x | x |
| Immunotherapy at this facility | | x | | | |
| Date other treatment started | x | | | | x |
| Other treatment | x | | | x | x |
| Other treatment at this facility | | x | | | |
| Protocol eligibility status | | x | | | |
| Protocol participation | | x | | | |
| **RECURRENCE** | | | | | |
| Date of first recurrence | x | | | | |
| Type of first recurrence | x | | | | |
| Other type of first recurrence(s) | | x | | | |
| Date(s) of subsequent treatment(s) for recurrence or progression | | x | | | |
| Type(s) of subsequent treatment for recurrence or progression | | x | | | |
| Recurrence site(s) | | | x | | |
| **FOLLOW-UP** | | | | | |
| Date of last contact or death | x | | | x | x |
| Vital status | x | | | x | x |
| Cancer status | x | | | | |

*Section Three: Comparison of Data Sets*

| ITEM | COC | | | SEER | NPCR |
|------|-----|---|---|------|------|
| | R | S | O | | |
| Quality of survival | | | x | | |
| Reconstruction/restoration-delayed | x | | | | * |
| Following registry | | | x | | |
| Follow-up source | | x | | | |
| Next follow-up source | | x | | | |
| Unusual follow-up method | | | x | | |
| Cause of death | | | x | x | x |
| ICD revision number | | | x | x | x |
| Autopsy | | | x | | |
| Commission on Cancer coding system - current | x | | | | |

# Index

## A

Access to care, 8, 9, 67, 109, 110, 120–122
    patient attitudes and, 48, 121
Accreditation of health care organizations,
        5–6, 27, 68–69, 84, 116, 125–126
Accreditation of insurance organizations,
        5–6, 27, 48, 68–69, 84, 116, 125–
        126
    National Committee for Quality As-
        surance (NCQA), 5, 48, 66–68, 83–
        84, 85, 86, 116
Accreditation of providers, 23, 27, 67,
        116, 125–126
Accountability, 1, 8, 9, 11, 18, 25, 66, 73,
        86, 94, 110, 111, 115, 125–126
    Foundation for Accountability
        (FACCT), 26, 36, 83, 85
Achievable Benchmarks of Care, 63
Adaptability, see Technological innova-
    tions (adaptability)
Adjuvant therapies, 59, 119
    breast cancer, 19, 25, 33, 81, 112,
        133, 136
    colon cancer, 32, 33, 47, 79
    see also Chemotherapy; Radiation
        therapy

African Americans, 59, 136
Age factors, 33, 65, 132–134 (*passim*),
        138, 139, 140, 146
    see also Elderly persons
Agency for Healthcare Research and
    Quality (AHRQ), 6, 7, 34, 44, 45,
        48, 49, 71, 84–85, 89, 90, 91, 92,
        117, 126
Aggregate quality scores, 3, 12, 16, 17,
        30, 46, 69, 71, 78
AIDS Cost and Services Utilization
    Study, 43
Ambulatory care, 3, 5, 6, 34, 43, 65, 85,
        88, 89, 118, 119, 142–143
American Association of Family Physi-
    cians, 85
American Cancer Society (ACS), 41–42,
        44, 58, 126
    see also National Cancer Data Base
American College of Physicians, 85
American College of Radiology, 20, 23–
        24
American College of Surgeons' Commis-
    sion on Cancer, 4, 31, 33, 116, 126
    see also National Cancer Data Base
American Diabetes Association, 85
American Indians, 59

American Medical Association, 66
American Society of Clinical Oncology
(ASCO), 22, 49, 83, 91
Attitudes and beliefs
patient satisfaction, *see* Patient satisfaction
patients, other, 48, 121
providers, general, 13, 29, 110
providers, toward elderly, 121–122
public opinion, 109, 110

**B**

Benchmarks, 3, 6, 9, 12, 16, 46, 48, 55, 63,
66, 75, 76, 78, 80, 81, 88, 90, 125
case studies, 21, 36
Biopsies, 25, 30, 47, 70, 112, 137
Black persons, *see* African Americans
Breast cancer, 12, 19, 41, 42, 63, 70, 92,
112, 120, 132–140
adjuvant therapies, 19, 25, 33, 81,
112, 133, 136
case studies, 19, 20, 21, 25–36 (*passim*), 79
diagnosis, not mammography, 12, 28,
30, 47, 50, 70, 112, 132–140
mammography, 28, 21, 43, 47, 51,
62–63, 66, 111, 112, 137
patient satisfaction, 25, 29, 51
quality-of-care measures, 47, 49, 50–
51, 83
radiation therapy, 25, 26, 27, 28, 31,
33, 47, 89, 112, 133, 134, 136, 139
surgery, 25, 26, 28, 30–31, 43, 44, 47,
50, 70, 81, 89, 112, 113, 132–140
survival rates and durations, 21, 26,
29, 139, 140
treatment, 12, 20, 39, 50, 79, 132,
133, 134; *see also "radiation therapy" and "surgery" supra*

**C**

Cancer Registries Amendment Act, 57, 72
Cancer Research Network, 42–43, 126
Case-control studies, 13
Case studies, 10, 18–36, 79, 80
benchmarks, 21, 36

breast cancer, 19, 20, 21, 25–36 (*passim*), 79
chemotherapy, 21, 22, 25, 26, 33
clinical practice guidelines, 19, 20,
21, 22, 23, 27, 30, 34–35, 79
colorectal cancer, 20, 24, 27, 31, 32–
33
comorbidity, 19, 27, 33
computer-based patient records, 19,
20, 22, 30, 79
diagnosis, 20, 21, 25, 28, 30, 34, 79
end-of-life care, 20, 21, 36, 79
health insurance, 20, 26–27, 28, 30–
31, 33, 34, 55, 79
hospitals and hospitalization, 21, 25,
33, 79
medical charts and records, 20, 23,
26, 28, 32–33, 34
outcome measures, 22, 23, 25, 26, 27
pain control, 21, 36
patient satisfaction, 21, 25, 26, 29, 34
performance standards, 22, 27, 28–29,
36
privacy and confidentiality, 27, 32–33
process standards, 23, 26
quality-of-care measures, 21, 24–26,
34, 36, 79
radiation therapy, 23–24, 24, 25, 26,
27, 28, 31, 33
registries, 20, 28, 29, 34
stages of cancer, 19, 25, 26–27, 28,
33, 34
treatment, general, 20, 21, 27, 79
Centers for Disease Control and Prevention (CDC), 4, 6, 85, 87, 89, 90, 121
*see also* National Program of Cancer
Registries
Cervical and uterine cancer, 24, 41, 42,
49, 63, 85, 121
Cervical Cancer Early Detection Program,
121
Charts, *see* Medical charts and records
Chemotherapy, 5, 12, 40, 41, 47, 48, 50,
81, 85, 112, 113, 134
case studies, 21, 22, 25, 26, 33
registries, 58
Clinical practice guidelines, 14, 80, 85,
90, 113–114, 133
case studies, 19, 20, 21, 22, 23, 27,
30, 34–35, 79

Clinical trials, 12, 13, 41, 43, 47, 81, 111, 116, 117
Cohort studies, 13, 15, 58
Colorectal cancer, 39, 40, 47, 49, 70, 92
    adjuvant therapies, 32, 33, 47, 79
    case studies, 20, 24, 27, 31, 32–33
    surgery, 33, 44, 70
Communications, 4, 14
    Intranets, 6, 14, 53, 90
    *see also* Internet
Comorbidity, 3, 6, 9, 40, 45, 48, 119
    case studies, 19, 27, 33
    registries, 58, 92, 135, 136, 140
    reporting standardized, 6, 12, 14, 19, 54–55, 77, 84, 85–86, 87, 90
    secondary (metastatic) cancer, 12, 53, 117
Computer-based patient records, 2, 3, 4, 6, 10, 12, 13–14, 38, 52–53, 75, 77, 80–81, 90, 93
    case studies, 19, 20, 22, 30, 79
    Intranets, 6, 14, 53, 90
    privacy and confidentiality, 4, 71, 73, 81, 93
Confidentiality, *see* Privacy and confidentiality
Consent, *see* Informed consent
Consumer Assessment of Health Plans Survey, 34
Cost factors, *see* Economic factors
Cross-sectional studies, 3, 12, 42, 46, 77

**D**

Demographic factors, 11, 33, 40, 57, 58, 59, 60, 118, 119, 120, 121
    socioeconomic status, 15, 40
    *see also* Age factors; Elderly persons; Geographic factors; Population-based studies; Race/ethnicity
Demonstration projects, 6, 7, 94
    *see also* Case studies
Department of Health and Human Services, 5–6, 43, 49, 73, 74, 84, 86, 93
    *see also* Agency for Healthcare Research and Quality; Centers for Disease Control and Prevention; Food and Drug Administration; Health Care Financing Administration;
    National Center for Health Statistics; National Institutes of Health
Department of Veterans Affairs, 6, 7, 38, 84–85, 90, 92
Diabetes, 52, 63, 85
Diagnosis, 4–5, 8, 9, 12, 39, 70, 92, 110, 114–115, 121
    biopsies, 25, 30, 47, 70, 112, 137
    breast cancer, 12, 28, 30, 47, 50, 70, 112, 132–140; *see also* Mammography
    case studies, 20, 21, 25, 28, 30, 34, 79
    cervical cancer, 121
    recently diagnosed patients, 1–2, 9, 15, 31, 42, 46, 76, 118, 119, 135
    registry data, 37–38, 40, 41, 42, 45, 92, 132–137
    secondary cancer, 12, 53, 117
    *see also* Stage of cancer
Drug treatment, *see* Chemotherapy; Medication

**E**

Economic factors, 2, 43, 52, 115
    costs of assessment, 19, 31, 59, 75, 80, 119, 127
    costs of care, 19, 21, 25, 38, 39, 44, 116, 120, 126, 134
    socioeconomic status, 15
    *see also* Funding; Health Care Financing Administration; Health insurance
Educational attainment, 121
Education and training
    funding, 23, 90, 119
    patient, 49, 69, 71, 112, 116, 117
    professional, 1, 22, 23, 52, 59, 67, 90, 94, 110, 119
Elderly persons, 39, 69, 92, 111, 115, 120, 121–122, 125, 132, 135, 136, 139
    Medicare, 32–33, 38, 39, 40, 43, 58, 69, 75, 87, 91, 93, 115, 118, 120, 125, 133, 135
Electronic Communications Privacy Act, 73
Electronic patient records, *see* Computer-based patient records

Employer-based health insurance, 31, 34,
    66, 71, 115
HEDIS, 48, 66–68, 89
End-of-life care, 8, 12, 39, 44, 51, 80, 117
    case studies, 20, 21, 36, 79
*Ensuring Quality Cancer Care*, 1, 8–10,
    48, 71, 76, 83, 91, 109
Ethnicity, *see* Race/ethnicity
Expert opinion, 13, 22, 23, 43, 81, 85, 90
    peer review organizations (PROs), 27,
    32, 69, 92, 125


**F**


Federal government, 2, 6–7, 18, 43–44,
    45, 49, 86, 89, 90–91, 94
    clinical trials, 117
    national data systems, 2, 11, 14–16,
    77, 86–88, 94, 111, 119
    privacy and confidentiality, 72, 74, 93
    *see also* Department of Health and
    Human Services; Department of
    Veterans Affairs; Funding; Legisla-
    tion
Fee-for-service plans, 33, 37, 38, 39, 40,
    119
Females, *see* Breast cancer; Cervical and
    uterine cancer; Gender factors
Food and Drug Administration, 6, 90
Foundation for Accountability (FACCT),
    26, 36, 83, 85
Freedom of Information Act, 72
Funding, 6–7, 18, 37, 43, 89, 119
    education and training, 23, 90, 119
    National Program of Cancer Regis-
    tries, 6, 7, 57, 61, 87, 88, 92–93
    peer review organizations, 92
    registries, 42, 57, 59, 88, 89


**G**


Gender factors, 33, 65, 132, 146
    *see also* Breast cancer; Cervical and
    uterine cancer; Prostate cancer
Geographic factors, 9, 11, 15, 16, 46, 57,
    59, 61, 65, 66, 77, 81, 82, 93, 115,
    125, 135, 146
    rural areas, 59, 138
    urban areas, 33, 65, 133, 138


**H**


Healthcare Cost and Utilization Project,
    44, 45
Health Care Financing Administration
    (HCFA), 6, 7, 63, 84–85, 88, 89, 92,
    115, 125
    case studies, 27, 32
    linkage studies, 7, 38, 57
    *see also* Medicaid; Medicare
Health insurance, 5, 9, 55, 69, 71, 77, 84,
    86, 93, 117, 120
    accreditation, 5–6, 27, 48, 68–69, 84,
    116, 125–126
    case studies, 20, 26–27, 28, 30–31,
    33, 34, 55, 79
    computer-based patient records, 53
    fee-for-service plans, 33, 37, 38, 39,
    40, 119
    registries, linkage to, 37–38, 40–42,
    45, 57–65 (*passim*), 71–72, 74, 91–
    93, 119, 135
    uninsured and underinsured persons,
    11, 15, 120, 139
    *see also* Employer-based health insur-
    ance; Managed care; Medicaid;
    Medicare
Health Insurance Portability and Ac-
    countability Act, 73, 74, 93
Health maintenance organizations, 33, 37,
    38, 39, 42–43, 67, 68, 126
*Healthy People 2010*, 56, 66
HEDIS (Health Plan Employer Data In-
    formation Set), 48, 66–68, 89
Hospice care, *see* End-of-life care
Hospitals and hospitalization, 38, 44, 69,
    125, 126
    benchmarks, 9, 63
    case studies, 21, 25, 33, 79
    hospital-based data retrieval, 3, 5, 6,
    89, 92, 133, 134, 138, 139, 140
    registries, 20, 25, 34, 38, 56(n.5), 58,
    60, 61, 65, 78, 79, 133, 134, 138,
    139, 140
    pain control, 21
    *see also* Medical charts and records


**I**


IMSystem, 69, 70

Independent Health Association, 30
Informed consent, 42, 45
Insurance, *see* Health insurance
International Association of Cancer Registries, 62
Internet, 2, 27, 48
  Agency for Health Research and Quality (AHRQ), 85
  computer-based patient records, 53
  Healthcare Cost and Utilization Project, 44
  HEDIS, 67
  Joint Commission for the Accreditation of Healthcare Organizations, 68
  National Center for Health Statistics, 44
  National Forum for Health Care Quality Measurement and Reporting, 52
  Quality Compass, 68
  Quality Interagency Coordination Task Force, 49
  SEER, 93
Intranets, 6, 14, 53, 90


**J**


Joint Commission for the Accreditation of Healthcare Organizations (JCAHO), 5–6, 33(n.1), 66, 68–69, 84, 86, 88, 126


**L**


Legal issues, 124
  informed consent, 42, 45
  malpractice, 137
  *see also* Privacy and confidentiality
Legislation
  Cancer Registries Amendment Act, 57, 72
  Electronic Communications Privacy Act, 73
  Freedom of Information Act, 72
  Health Insurance Portability and Accountability Act, 73, 74, 93
  Privacy Act, 72
Linkage studies, 7, 37–39, 40–42, 45, 57–65 (*passim*), 71–72, 74, 78, 91–93, 119, 133–136

Health Care Financing Administration (HCFA), 7, 38, 57
  health insurance, 37–38, 40–42, 45, 57–65 (*passim*), 71–72, 74, 91–93, 119, 135
  National Cancer Institute, 7, 34, 37–39
  SEER, 7, 38–39, 41, 45, 57, 62–63, 87, 91, 92–93, 118
Local systems of care, 12, 16, 42, 46, 66–75, 92, 125
  case studies, 20–22
  *see also* Health insurance; Hospitals and hospitalization; Provider groups
Lung cancer, 21, 39, 44, 47, 49, 70, 81, 85, 120, 135


**M**


Males, *see* Gender factors; Prostate cancer
Malpractice, 137
Mammography, 28, 21, 43, 47, 51, 62–63, 66, 111, 112, 137
Managed care, 40, 42–43, 45, 48–49, 68, 80–81, 119, 126
  benchmarks, 9
  case studies, 26, 30
  geographic variation, 15
  National Committee for Quality Assurance (NCQA), 5, 48, 66–68, 83–84, 85, 86, 116
  *see also* Health insurance; Health maintenance organizations
Medicaid, 69, 115, 139
Medical charts and records, 3, 5, 12, 40, 54–55, 78, 79, 80, 92, 112
  case studies, 20, 23, 26, 28, 32–33, 34
  *see also* Computer-based patient records; Privacy and confidentiality
Medical Expenditure Panel Survey, 43
Medicare, 32–33, 38, 39, 40, 43, 58, 69, 75, 87, 91, 93, 115, 118, 120, 125, 133, 135
Medication, 19, 23, 27, 40, 43, 63, 113, 120, 132, 133, 138, 140
  *see also* Chemotherapy; Pain and pain control (palliative care)
MEDSTAT, 69
Men, *see* Gender factors; Prostate cancer
Minority groups, *see* Race/ethnicity

Models and modeling, 6, 85
  see also Case studies; Demonstration
  projects

**N**

National Ambulatory Medical Care Survey, 43
National Cancer Data Base (NCDB), 4, 6,
  31, 55, 59–62 (*passim*), 65, 71–72,
  74, 82, 87, 88, 89, 90, 118, 125,
  148–154
National Cancer Institute (NCI), 23, 42,
  45, 48, 71, 75, 83, 84, 87, 89, 91,
  117
  educational efforts, 7, 23
  demonstration projects, 7
  funding, 6, 7, 59
  linkage studies, 7, 34, 37–39
  registries, general, 4, 38, 39, 40, 41,
  92; see also Surveillance, Epidemiology, and End Results (SEER)
  program
National Center for Health Statistics, 44,
  59, 126
National Committee for Quality Assurance (NCQA), 5, 48, 66–68, 83–84,
  85, 86, 116
National Comprehensive Cancer Network
  (NCCN), 26, 27, 30, 35, 81, 84
National Coordinating Council for Cancer
  Surveillance, 62
National Death Index, 57
National Forum for Health Care Quality
  Measurement and Reporting, 49,
  52, 86
National Health Interview Survey, 43
National Home and Hospice Care Survey,
  44
National Hospital Discharge Survey, 44
National Institutes of Health, 6, 90
  see also National Cancer Institute
National Mortality Followback Survey, 44
National Program of Cancer Registries
  (NPCR), 4, 39, 55, 56–64 (*passim*),
  71–72, 74, 82, 87, 89, 123, 148–154
  funding, 6, 7, 57, 61, 87, 88, 92–93
Nationwide Inpatient Sample, 44
Native Americans, see American Indians

North American Association of Central
  Cancer Registries, 56, 62, 146–147

**O**

Organizational factors, 1, 15, 112, 127
  accreditation of health care organizations, 5–6, 27, 33(n.1), 68–69, 84,
  116, 125–126
  provider practice management, 19,
  22, 34, 79, 80
  research consortiums, 37, 42–43, 45,
  93, 114
Outcome measures, 2, 12, 14, 41, 44, 47,
  48, 110, 112, 118, 119, 121
  case studies, 22, 23, 25, 26, 27
  computer-based patient records, 46
  registries, 37, 58
  see also Quality of life; Survival rates
  and durations
Outpatient care, see Ambulatory care

**P**

Pain and pain control (palliative care), 2,
  8, 12, 16, 44, 50, 51, 80, 110, 117
  case studies, 21, 36
  see also End-of-life care
Patient attitudes and beliefs, general, 48,
  121
  see also Patient satisfaction
Patient education, 49, 69, 71, 112, 116,
  117
  educational attainment of patients,
  121
Patient records, see Computer-based patient records; Medical charts and records
Patient satisfaction, 13, 40–41, 67, 71, 80,
  110, 115–116, 119
  breast cancer patients, 25, 29, 51
  case studies, 21, 25, 26, 29, 34
  end-of-life care, 21
  see also Quality of life
Patterns of care studies, 23–24, 81
Peer review organizations (PROs), 27, 32,
  69, 92, 125
Performance standards, 1, 6, 48, 69, 78,
  80, 85, 86, 94, 135

case studies, 22, 27, 28–29, 36
  *see also* Benchmarks; Outcome
  measures
Pharmaceuticals, *see* Medication
Political factors, 1
Population-based studies, 3, 12, 14–16,
  45, 46, 55–63, 77, 81–82, 87, 88,
  126, 142–145
  cohort studies, 13, 15, 58
  mammography, 63, 66
  workshop agenda, 123–124
  *see also* Demographic factors; National Cancer Data Base; National
  Program of Cancer Registries; Registries; Surveillance, Epidemiology,
  and End Results (SEER) program
Poverty, *see* Socioeconomic status
President's Advisory Commission on Consumer Protection and Quality in the
  Health Care Industry, 49, 86, 114
Preventive Services Task Force, 13
Privacy Act, 72
Privacy and confidentiality, 3, 4, 7, 12,
  45, 46, 71–75, 77, 94
  case studies, 27, 32–33
  computer-based records, 4, 71, 73, 81,
  93
  legislation, 72, 73, 74, 93
  registries, 71–72, 73, 74, 93, 124
  state government, 73, 74–75, 92
Process standards, 12, 13, 37, 46, 48, 66,
  77, 80, 112, 118
  case studies, 23, 26
  *see also* Benchmarks
Professional education and training, 1, 22,
  23, 52, 59, 67, 90, 94, 110, 119
PROs, *see* Peer review organizations
Prostate cancer, 24, 31, 39, 41, 42, 45, 47,
  49, 60, 85, 113, 133, 136
  surgery, 45, 85, 133
Provider groups, 9, 16, 19–23, 25, 34
Public opinion, 109, 110

**Q**

Q-SPAN, 85
Quality Compass, 68
Quality Interagency Coordination Task
  Force, 49, 86

Quality-of-case measures, 2, 5, 40, 51, 61,
  67, 77, 78, 83–86, 109, 111–118,
  119–120, 124
  adaptability, 3, 17
  aggregate quality scores, 3, 12, 16,
  17, 30, 46, 69, 71, 78
  case studies, 21, 24–26, 34, 36, 79
  core set, 5–6, 12–13, 36, 46, 47–52,
  114–116
  discrete populations, 16
  lacking, 3, 19, 75, 80, 81, 83
  risk-adjusted, 39
  time-series analysis, 3, 13, 16, 23–24
  workshop agenda, 123
  *see also* Accountability; Benchmarks;
  Outcome measures; Performance
  standards; Process standards; Standards, general
Quality of life, 25, 27, 29, 41, 44, 45, 111
  *see also* End-of-life care

**R**

Race/ethnicity, 11, 24, 33, 59, 60, 65,
  120, 121, 132, 133, 136, 140, 146
  African Americans, 59, 136
  American Indians, 59
  language factors, 67
Radiation therapy, 5, 24, 26, 40, 119, 133
  American College of Radiology, 20,
  23–24
  breast cancer, 25, 26, 27, 28, 31, 33,
  47, 89, 112, 133, 134, 136, 139
  case studies, 23–24, 24, 25, 26, 27,
  28, 31, 33
RAND, 91
Records, *see* Computer-based patient
  records; Medical charts and records;
  Privacy and confidentiality
Registries, 3, 5, 39–42, 61, 77, 78, 87–89,
  91–92
  administrative data and, 37–39
  case studies, 20, 28, 29, 34
  comorbidity, 58, 92, 135, 136, 140
  computer-based patient records, 14, 53
  diagnosis, 37–38, 40, 41, 42, 45, 92,
  132–137
  funding, 42, 57, 59, 88, 89

health insurance records and, 37–38, 40–42, 45, 57–65 (*passim*), 71–72, 74, 91–93, 119, 135

hospital, 20, 25, 34, 38, 56(n.5), 58, 60, 61, 65, 78, 79, 133, 134, 138, 139, 140

linkage efforts, 7, 37–39, 40–42, 45, 57–65 (*passim*), 71–72, 74, 91–93, 119, 133–136

National Cancer Institute, general, 4, 38, 39, 40, 41, 92; *see also* Surveillance, Epidemiology, and End Results (SEER) program

North American Association of Central Cancer Registries, 56, 62, 146–147

outcome measures, 37, 58

privacy and confidentiality, 71–72, 73, 74, 93, 124

special studies, 37, 39, 41–42, 45, 87, 91–92

stage of cancer, 37, 40, 45, 58, 84, 92, 136, 139

standards, general, 39, 57, 59, 64, 146–147

state government role, 5, 6, 20, 32–33, 39, 40–42, 45, 56–60, 64–65, 72, 74–75, 84, 88, 91–93

indicators of data quality, by state, 142–146

individual state studies, 132–140

survival rates, 58, 65, 139, 140

workshop agenda, 123–124

*see also* National Cancer Data Base; National Program of Cancer Registries

Reporting requirements, 3, 6, 14, 15, 17, 53–55, 79, 112

aggregate quality scores, 3, 12, 16, 17, 30, 46, 69, 71, 78

comorbidity, standards, 6, 12, 14, 19, 54–55, 77, 84, 85–86, 87, 90

stage of cancer, standards, 3, 6, 12, 14, 19, 46, 53–54, 77, 84, 85–86, 90

standards, general, 3, 14, 39, 69, 75, 77, 79, 80

treatment, standards, 20, 46, 87

*see also* Computer-based patient records; Registries

Risk factors, 39, 42, 43, 49

smoking, 42, 43, 63, 117

Rural areas, 59, 138

**S**

Sampling, 15–16, 24, 41, 43, 44, 49, 83

Secondary (metastatic) cancer, 12, 53, 117

SEER, *see* Surveillance, Epidemiology, and End Results (SEER) program

Skin cancer, 41, 49, 53, 60

Smoking, 42, 43, 63, 117

Socioeconomic status, 15, 40, 65, 77, 119, 132, 133, 134, 140, 146

Medicaid, 69, 115, 139

Special studies, 6, 37, 39, 41–42, 45, 87, 91–92

Stage of cancer, 12, 15, 42, 43, 44, 50, 70, 113, 119

case studies, 19, 25, 26–27, 28, 33, 34

recently diagnosed patients, 1–2, 9, 15, 31, 42, 46, 76, 118, 119, 135

registry data, 37, 40, 45, 58, 84, 92, 136, 139

reporting standardized, 3, 6, 12, 14, 19, 46, 53–54, 77, 84, 85–86, 90

secondary (metastatic) cancer, 12, 53, 117

Standards, general, 13, 18, 21, 43, 73, 110

accreditation of health care organizations, 5–6, 27, 33(n.1), 68–69, 84, 116, 125–126

accreditation of insurance organizations, 5–6, 27, 48, 68–69, 84, 116, 125–126

National Committee for Quality Assurance (NCQA), 5, 48, 66–68, 83–84, 85, 86, 116

accreditation of providers, 23, 27, 67, 116, 125–126

computer-based records, 13–14, 80–81

quality of life, 25, 27, 29, 41, 44, 45, 111

registries, 39, 57, 59, 64, 146–147

*see also* Benchmarks; Clinical practice guidelines; Outcome measures; Performance standards; Process standards; Quality-of-care measures; Reporting requirements

State government, 2, 4, 15, 16

Medicaid, 69, 115
peer review organizations (PROs), 27, 32, 69, 92, 125
privacy and confidentiality, 73, 74–75, 92
registries, 5, 6, 20, 32–33, 39, 40–42, 45, 56–60, 64–65, 72, 74–75, 84, 88, 91–93
  indicators of data quality, by state, 142–146
  individual state studies, 132–140
  *see also* National Cancer Data Base; National Program of Cancer Registries; Surveillance, Epidemiology, and End Results (SEER) program
State Inpatient Database, 44
Statistical analyses, 13, 15, 49, 136
  aggregate quality scores, 3, 12, 16, 17, 30, 46, 69, 71, 78
  case-control studies, 13
  clinical trials, 12, 13, 41, 43, 47, 81, 111, 116, 117
  cohort studies, 13, 15, 58
  cross-sectional studies, 3, 12, 42, 46, 77
  sampling, 15–16, 24, 41, 43, 44, 49, 83
  time-series analysis, 3, 13, 16, 23–24
Supportive care, 9, 20, 43
Surgery, 44, 70, 113, 135, 142–143
  breast cancer, 25, 26, 28, 30–31, 43, 44, 47, 50, 70, 81, 89, 112, 113, 132–140
  colon cancer, 33, 44, 70
  prostate cancer, 45, 85, 133
Surveillance, 118–119
  *see also* National Cancer Data Base; National Program of Cancer Registries; Registries; Reporting requirements; Surveillance, Epidemiology, and End Results (SEER) program
Surveillance, Epidemiology, and End Results (SEER) program, 4, 6, 45, 55, 59–65 (*passim*), 82, 87, 88, 89, 93, 124, 136, 146, 148–154
  linkage efforts, 7, 38–39, 41, 45, 57, 62–63, 87, 91, 92–93, 118
Survival rates and durations, 21, 23, 39, 40, 42, 55, 59, 111, 113, 119
  breast cancer, 21, 26, 29, 139, 140
  registries, 58, 65, 139, 140
Survivorship issues, 43, 44, 45, 116–117, 126

**T**

Technological innovations (adaptability), 3, 5, 12, 17, 46, 78
  *see also* Computer-based patient records; Internet; Intranets
Telecommunications, 4
  Intranets, 6, 14, 53, 90
  *see also* Internet
Time-series analysis, 3, 13, 16
  Patterns of care studies, 23–24
Tobacco use, *see* Smoking
Training, *see* Education and training
Treatment, 4–5, 9, 12, 40, 43, 44, 58, 85, 110, 111, 113, 118
  breast cancer, 12, 20, 39, 50, 79, 132, 133, 134
  case studies, 20, 21, 27, 79
  clinical trials, 12, 13, 41, 43, 47, 81, 111, 116, 117
  elderly persons, 121–122, 132, 135, 136, 139
  provider groups, 20, 21
  reporting standardized, 20, 46, 87
  *see also* Adjuvant therapies; Chemotherapy; Medication; Pain and pain control (palliative care); Radiation therapy; Surgery

**U**

Uninsured and underinsured persons, 11, 15, 120, 139
Urban areas, 33, 65, 133, 138

**V**

Veterans Affairs, *see* Department of Veterans Affairs

**W**

Women, *see* Breast cancer; Cervical and uterine cancer; Gender factors
World Wide Web, *see* Internet